# Parenting ADHD NOW!

ELAINE TAYLOR-KLAUS &
DIANE DEMPSTER

# Parenting ADHD NOW!

## Easy Intervention Strategies to Empower Kids with ADHD

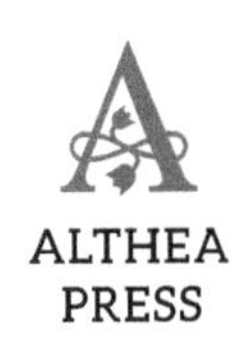

ALTHEA
PRESS

For general information on our other products and services or to obtain technical support, please contact our Customer Care Department within the United States at (866) 744-2665, or outside the United States at (510) 253-0500.

Althea Press publishes its books in a variety of electronic and print formats. Some content that appears in print may not be available in electronic books, and vice versa.



ISBN: Print 978-1-62315-782-1 | eBook 978-1-62315-783-8

# Contents

# Introduction

Children with Attention Deficit/Hyperactivity Disorder (ADHD) have a whole industry of committed professionals working diligently to improve their lives. If all goes well, these psychologists, therapists, coaches, tutors, special educators, and occupational therapists, among others, teach children with ADHD how to learn, how to understand their brain's unique wiring, and how to manage themselves so they can grow to become successful adults.

But what about the parents of children with ADHD? Who is focused on supporting *you*? Who is teaching you what you need to understand about your child? Who is helping you learn how to be the best parent you can be for a child whose ADHD complicates childhood—and parenting? Who is helping you figure out how to apply the experts' advice to your family when one kid is bouncing off the walls and another one is melting down, the pot is boiling over on the stove, the counters are too cluttered to find anything, and homework hasn't even been started?

Parental options for support tend to be limited to therapy, consulting, and information gathering. But you know you need something more, something to sustain you and prevent you from feeling isolated. There are plenty of resources telling you what to do. But what's missing is the resources telling you *how*. How do you manage this complicated child in a way that works for your whole family?

## Who Are We?

We are Diane Dempster and Elaine Taylor-Klaus, parents, coaches, educators, and the cofounders of ImpactADHD. We started off just like you. But in a few short years, we have become national leaders in the world of ADHD, representatives of the voice of parents, and the go-to experts for parenting children with ADHD. But that's not what truly qualifies us to write this book—or why you should read it. You'll want to read this book because:

- We understand the experience of parenting, living with, and raising kids with ADHD . . . because we are living it.
- We understand that parents of kids with ADHD are stretched too thin in terms of time and money . . . because we are, too.
- We know you need support that is effective, affordable, accessible, and practical . . . because we need it, too.
- Most of all, we understand you have no time to waste and you're afraid that time will pass too quickly before you figure out how to manage (dare we say, master?) your child's ADHD . . . and we are right there with you.

In 2010, we met each other at a Children and Adults with ADHD (CHADD) conference in Atlanta, Georgia. Back then, we were just two moms who happened to be coaches, trying to make sense of our complicated worlds. We discovered we had three things in common:

1. We shared a frustration over how little guidance and training were available specifically for parents of children with ADHD. Between our families, we had six kids and two spouses with ADHD and related challenges. As we sought answers, and ways to understand and manage the ADHD in our homes, there was not much available to help us navigate the choppy waters. We appreciated that CHADD provided essential information about ADHD, and that some parents were lucky enough to live in a community with a strong local support group (or were organized enough to start one). But we needed something that was not readily available for parents—something that went beyond information and hand-holding.

2. We discovered that as certified professional coaches, challenged with managing ADHD in our own families, we had become much better parents to our kids with ADHD when each of us became a coach. In our professional practices, we guided clients to greater clarity and helped them remove obstacles to success and satisfaction in their lives. Through coaching, we learned to set realistic, attainable goals and communicate fundamental components of effective parenting. Coaching empowered us to bring those skills to our parenting approach. It made a world of difference, and we realized we could teach it to other parents.
3. We discovered we had each worked in some aspect of health care all of our professional lives: Elaine primarily as an advocate and educator, and Diane as an administrator and educator. Because we had each worked on the national level, we looked at the need for change from a big-picture perspective. We understood clearly that parents are the missing link in ADHD management and that they need more than information and guidance to be the best advocates they can be for their child's health care.

## The Challenge and the Opportunity

Raising children with ADHD is messy and complicated, and can be unbelievably frustrating for parents—whether we have ADHD ourselves (which is true for Elaine) or not. Something needed to be done to reduce parents' stress and improve the outcomes for their kids. So we joined forces to create ImpactADHD, determined to fill a critical void: to focus on serving the needs of parents of children with ADHD.

We were determined to give parents something they were missing: expert guidance that focuses on the reality of living with ADHD challenges. Immediately, we struck a chord. We were selected by CHADD as an Innovative Program in 2011, and we launched our first website at the CHADD conference later that year. In less than two years, ImpactADHD was presenting at national conferences and supporting parents in more than 100 countries each month with articles, coaching tips, webinars, products, and services. We are now featured in many videos and on numerous websites, and have delivered workshops for parents and teachers all over the world. There's more information about us and ImpactADHD in the back of the book.

## What This Book Offers

This book is not a parent's primer for ADHD—many sources cover the basics, such as the ImpactADHD and CHADD websites. In this book, we offer guidance that combines effective techniques with what we call a "coach-approach" to parenting. We will teach you to use strategies that build confidence and improve communication, as well as get the homework turned in. It's not enough to tell you *what* to do—we will give you a context in which to begin to do it more effectively.

We will not promise that you'll get absolutely everything you need out of this book—we have been sold that bag of goods ourselves! While we offer real hope grounded in proven strategies, there is no magic bullet or cure. This book assumes you understand that ADHD is a lifelong condition (for most) to be managed—consciously and effectively.

We *will* promise that, with this book, you will be better able to set limits, try new things, find acceptance, change your habits, laugh instead of cry, and understand instead of yell—thrive instead of just survive. You will learn strategies for effective management, tools to confidently minimize ADHD-related stress in your family, and suggestions to foster independence and success in your children.

This book is different from other ADHD-strategy books in three ways: (1) it is grounded in the coach-approach to parenting, (2) it offers practical strategies for the real lives of families with ADHD, and (3) it focuses on you—the parent—more than on your child.

We know you can dramatically improve life for your child with ADHD. We know you can manage the roller coaster of raising your ADHD kid—and we want to help you enjoy the ride! As a parent, you are so used to giving to others that, all too often, you have nothing left for yourself. Empowering yourself is the best way to empower your child—and that is what we aim to help you accomplish.

PART ONE

# The Highlights

CHAPTER 1

# A Different Way of Being

If you have a child with ADHD in your life—whether you are raising, teaching, or otherwise supporting her—then you know that it's not a one-size-fits-all diagnosis. It's complicated. Sometimes *really* complicated.

A key point in understanding ADHD is that not all ADHD looks alike. ADHD presents differently in everyone who has it, which is part of what makes it so difficult to diagnose (or even accept). And while it tends to come with a balanced dose of strengths and challenges, the strengths can be difficult to grasp in the early stages of management, while the challenges can be bright and bold and easy for all to see.

The book offers strategies to make life with ADHD easier and more enjoyable. We won't spend a lot of time telling you what you already know, but we do think it's important to review some critical highlights of ADHD. In recent years, there have been some major changes in the way the medical community defines and describes ADHD, and it's important to better understand what it takes to manage ADHD in reality, not just in theory.

## The Faces of ADHD

Before we get into the current medical state of affairs around ADHD and the set of cognitive processes called *executive function*, let's take a moment to put a human face on the issue. Like snowflakes, no two people with ADHD have exactly the same experience. The intensity and specifics of a person's ADHD show up in many different behaviors and to different extents.

Several leading characteristics are used to define or describe common problem behaviors for people with ADHD—behaviors caused by a neurodevelopmental disorder. It's important to remember that these challenges are overlapping. Most children are challenged with several, if not all, of these behaviors. Typically, people with ADHD have trouble regulating or controlling five key aspects of behavior:

- Attention
- Hyperactivity
- Impulsivity
- Organization
- Emotionality

So let's get a better understanding of the complexity of each of these challenges and how each might present for children. Remember, there are varying degrees of challenge for each child, and sometimes these challenges change day by day. Look for what's familiar, but don't expect it to match your child precisely (though that could happen, too).

## ATTENTION

It is commonly assumed that ADHD is about not being able to pay attention. In reality, it's more accurate to say that the real challenge for people with ADHD is regulating attention, or the ability to manage attention. Managing attention goes far beyond limiting distractions. It is about being able to recognize what is important to focus attention on, being able to focus on it at the correct time, being able to shift attention from one thing to another, and being able to stop paying attention or focusing on something when it's time to do something else.

### *How Attention Challenges Present*

Peppermint Patty of *Peanuts* is often characterized as a D student, and she certainly seemed to struggle with attention issues. She had a difficult time paying attention to the teacher (rather than to Woodstock out on the windowsill or the kid tapping a pencil at the next desk), she was often confused about what action was required of her, and she rarely heard what her teacher said the first time. We can imagine that she struggled to shift her focus when her teacher changed subjects, and may have even had a difficult time stopping once she finally got into an assignment—unless it was time for the class to line up for recess. That's a lot more complicated than just paying attention, right?

Cookie Monster of *Sesame Street* has a hard time thinking about anything but cookies! He is a good example of how children with attention challenges can get stuck on one thing and find it hard to redirect to something else. This is often referred to as *hyperfocusing*. Much like many of our kids these days with video games, Cookie Monster finds it challenging to care much about anything else—which makes it particularly difficult for him to find the motivation to shift his attention away from the cookies when such a shift is expected of him.

## HYPERACTIVITY

It is commonly assumed that a hyperactive child with ADHD is always bouncing off the walls. Certainly, sometimes our kids move like they are powered by a supercharged battery, but it is important to understand that this experience is both external and internal. It's not just the physical body a child needs to learn to calm. In actuality, their challenge is learning to manage or regulate an overactive brain. World-renowned ADHD expert Dr. Ned Hallowell describes the difficulty as a "Ferrari brain with bicycle brakes." Among its other effects, a racing brain can cause difficulty sleeping, and just imagine what happens when a racing body tries to function without enough sleep.

### *How Hyperactivity Challenges Present*

Imagine Calvin from *Calvin and Hobbes* in the doctor's office. Some part of him knows that he's supposed to sit quietly while his mom talks to the doctor, but pretty soon he's sliding off the couch, and turning upside down with his head on the ground and his feet in the air. After trying to ignore Calvin, his mom finally gets aggravated (or embarrassed) and asks him to sit up. The doctor turns her attention to Calvin, who recognizes that all eyes are on him and it's time for him to start talking. He has no clue what to say because he wasn't paying attention, so he starts talking about all the things he's been thinking about for the eternity that the adults were talking (four minutes, at least!). He verbalizes the rapid-fire thoughts in his mind, chattering away about school, a recent adventure with Hobbes, the ride there, and what he wants for dinner. When redirected, he answers the doctor's questions. A moment after the adults start talking to each other again, he's sliding along the floor like a lizard in pursuit of a mosquito on the windowsill.

## IMPULSIVITY

Impulsive kids are often seen as rude and disrespectful, and even aggressive. In truth, these kids are facing a much more complex challenge than just trying to be nice: their brain wiring makes it difficult to control themselves in the moment. In a way, they are locked in the present without the capacity to think ahead. Before taking action, they can't easily think through what the consequences might be or what "later" might bring. We joke that people with ADHD have two time frames: now and not now. There's no "ready, get set, go" with these kids. It's "go, go, go!" With no consideration of future outcomes or consequences, and no ability to learn from past mistakes, they miss critical social cues, cause endless interruptions, and get physically hurt more often than their peers.

### *How Impulsivity Challenges Present*

Hammie is the precocious brother in the *Baby Blues* comic strip. His impulsivity creates a lot of friction at home, especially with his older sister. He is constantly interrupting conversations, messing up his sister's games, dropping dishes and breaking toys, saying hurtful things, and getting himself into precarious situations, like running into the street or climbing on the roof. He is not yet able to learn from his mistakes, and his exhausted mother feels like she can never safely leave him alone for an instant, much less with a babysitter. He can be charming and adorable, but the underlying lack of restraint is exhausting for all those around him.

## ORGANIZATION

Exploding backpacks and cluttered rooms are the hallmarks of children with ADHD who struggle with organization. Organization requires conscious self-management and some planning. This is not easy for children who struggle with distractibility, hyperactivity, and/or impulse control. When you don't know how to plan, prioritize, or sequence what needs to be done, it's difficult to keep on top of things—and it influences every aspect of life. It's not just about keeping track of things; it also presents as trouble keeping track of time and responsibilities, and even difficulty with the basics of self-care like hygiene, eating, and taking medications. The accompanying difficulty with reliability and follow-through also causes challenges in relationships.

### *How Organization Challenges Present*

Remember Jeremy from the comic strip *Zits*? Many strips feature the mess in his bedroom; clothes, papers, dishes, and random items are scattered everywhere. From the looks of this mess, we can imagine that Jeremy's disorganization probably started well before he became a teenager. His clutter probably wasn't limited to his room, either. At school, in the neighborhood, and around the house, he was likely always losing things. His parents might've needed to replace his winter coat twice in fourth grade, and those tests he was supposed to get signed never seemed to make it home for his parents to see. He didn't start brushing his teeth regularly until he had a girlfriend and his parents never really believed he'd be able to hold down a job. Frankly, they weren't sure he'd ever find his way out of the eighth grade.

## EMOTIONALITY

The connection between ADHD and what we call *emotional intensity* is a fairly new development in ADHD awareness. We now understand that managing emotions is a critical component of our executive skills, which tend to be developmentally delayed in kids with ADHD. Mood management is necessary to handle life's disappointments with some degree of decorum and to build strong relationships. But frustration intolerance is a key marker of ADHD, and these kids have a harder time handling disappointment than other kids. Of course, they experience disappointment more often than other kids do. With all of their impulsivity, inattention, hyperactivity, and disorganization, the adults in their lives tend to correct them—a lot! Over time, it impacts their self-esteem and their relationships with others.

### *How Mood Challenges Present*

Let's face it: Daffy Duck from *Looney Tunes* comics was never a very good sport. He always wanted things to go a certain way and threw tantrums when they didn't. He was disappointed a lot, for sure. After all, it's hard to be constantly bested by a smooth-talking bunny. But he also never handled it very well when things didn't lean in his favor, and he was absolutely unable to be wrong or admit his mistakes. Like Daffy, kids who struggle with emotional intensity overreact and take things personally, creating scenes and hijacking situations, making it difficult for parents to find compassion in the heat of embarrassment. "I'm always walking on eggshells" or "I never know what's going to set him off" are common refrains for parents of kids who struggle with emotional intensity.

## COEXISTING CONDITIONS

According to the Centers for Disease Control and Prevention (CDC), at least 20 percent of American children suffer from some form of mental disorder or "serious changes in the ways children handle their emotions, learn, or behave." This does not include other chronic conditions common in childhood, such as allergies.

According to the American Academy of Pediatrics, ADHD is one of the most commonly diagnosed conditions in childhood today, second only to asthma. And data from the CDC states that 11 percent (6.4 million) of school-age children in the United States have been diagnosed with ADHD, a number that increased 42 percent between 2003 and 2015. ADHD rarely exists alone in a child. In fact, more than two out of three (86 percent) of children diagnosed with ADHD have at least one other medical condition—such as anxiety, depression, an autism spectrum disorder, bipolar disorder, learning disabilities, asthma, allergies, celiac disease, juvenile diabetes, and Tourette syndrome. None of these conditions are adequately treated with medication alone; all require parent management (such as using the strategies in this book) as part of effective treatment.

The following are common coexisting conditions in children with ADHD:

Anxiety
Bipolar disorder
Conduct disorder
Depression
Learning disabilities
Oppositional defiant disorder

Other disorders have ADHD as a common coexisting condition:

Autism spectrum disorders
Sleep disorders and bed-wetting
Tourette syndrome

When seeking treatment for children with ADHD, it's important to identify other potential coexisting conditions. If you are concerned your child might be suffering from other conditions, ask your medical practitioner to assist you in exploring further evaluation. It is common for untreated ADHD, or ADHD that is not yet well managed, to look a lot like anxiety or depression. Consult a professional to help you determine what is really going on with your child.

Above all, trust your instincts. If you are well informed and well educated, if you understand your child's challenges and are getting support in learning how to manage them effectively, then you should be seeing positive improvement (not perfection, but progress). If you are not seeing improvements and have a sense something else is going on, you are probably right. Pursue it relentlessly until you get the support you need for your child. Don't give up hope—keep searching, asking questions, and most important, asking for help. There is no shame in asking for help raising complex children. Plus, asking for guidance is a critical skill to model for our kids.

## The New World of the ADHD Diagnosis—the Subtypes Redefined

ADHD is a neurodevelopmental disorder, meaning it affects how the nervous system works in relation to brain development. Here are a few distinctions we know about the brains of people with ADHD:

- People with ADHD often experience delays in the development of several areas of the brain, including the frontal lobe (the brain's "conductor").
- Brain structure and chemistry contribute to ADHD behaviors, and they are influenced by a variety of factors, including nature and nurture factors.
- The neurotransmitters in an ADHD brain do not work efficiently. When a message is sent from one part of the brain to another, it can get scrambled or directed to the wrong place, making it difficult for a person to move from idea to action.

These three things impact an individual's ability to self-regulate, which means that the brains of people with ADHD are not automatically wired well for self-control or self-management.

In 2013, the fifth edition of the *Diagnostic and Statistical Manual of Mental Disorders (DSM-5)* was released. The *DSM-5* presents a new framework that redefines the nuances of ADHD. Many parents today still think of ADHD in terms of the old framework and try to make a distinction between ADD and ADHD, using ADD to refer to inattentive type ADHD. Technically, while the terms are still sometimes used interchangeably, according to medical diagnostic criteria, ADHD is the proper term for all aspects of this condition:

- Inattentive type (formerly called ADD): challenged by distractibility and focus management
- Hyperactive type: challenged by excess energy and impulsivity
- Combined type: challenged by aspects of both types

In his article "What Parents of ADD/ADHD Kids Should Know (About the *DSM-5*)," developmental pediatrician Mark Bertin states, "The *DSM-5* removes the concept of ADHD subtypes (such as inattentive versus hyperactive). Instead, it describes 'predominant' symptoms (e.g., *ADHD with predominantly hyperactive features, or ADHD with predominantly inattentive features*) and rates severity (mild to severe)." This is not just an academic distinction. Removing the subtypes supports individuals more effectively, since they do not have exactly the same ADHD and it is likely to change over time.

In the new framework, Bertin says, "Diagnosis is based on observable, real-life behaviors because physical tests (such as brain scans or computer tests) and neuropsychological testing do not yet accurately identify ADHD on their own. The *DSM-5* broadens symptom explanations, helping providers recognize the wide range of ways ADHD reveals itself."

So, what does this mean for parents in terms of understanding your child's ADHD? Simply put, according to Bertin, "In spite of its name, ADHD is no longer seen as a disorder of attention, hyperactivity, or impulsivity alone. These symptoms occur as part of a larger umbrella of difficulties in executive function, representing all the cognitive abilities used to manage our lives, plan, and self-regulate."

## The Six Areas of Executive Functioning

It is difficult to understand ADHD without having some understanding of what is meant by the term *executive function*. Executive function is the set of organizing thoughts, feelings, and actions of the brain—which acts like the "orchestra conductor" of the brain. For people with ADHD, sometimes the brain is like an orchestra without a conductor.

Some people believe that ADHD should be described in terms of executive function deficits. Not only will looking at it this way help you as a parent better understand the nuances of your child's ADHD, but it will provide direction for you to identify strategies that can specifically address the five key challenging behaviors identified earlier.

Six aspects of executive function are commonly impaired (or delayed) in people with ADHD, which are described in the following sections. This information is drawn from research by clinical psychologist Thomas E. Brown and terminology used by Dr. Mark Bertin.

## TASK MANAGEMENT (ACTIVATION)

*Prioritizing, Organizing, and Initiating Activity*

**What it looks like:** Difficulty getting started, procrastinating, knowing what needs to be done but can't initiate tasks, difficulty prioritizing and sequencing, and failure in time management. People with activation issues may seem to have only two time frames: now and not now. They often get things done at the last minute, once it becomes now. Rather than initiating an activity from desire or intention, the activity gets done reactively because adrenaline from fear sets things in motion.

**Pros:** Ability to respond well in high-pressure situations, flexibility, responsiveness to new opportunities, and a tendency toward spontaneity.

**Cons:** Can appear lazy or disrespectful. Leads to disorganization.

## ATTENTION MANAGEMENT (FOCUS)

*Focusing, Sustaining, and Shifting Attention to Tasks*

**What it looks like:** Easily bored, requiring genuine interest in something to sustain focus; easily distracted, difficulty determining what is important to pay attention to; hyperfocus, locking in with intense diligence (as in video games); and unable to move off of task.

**Pros:** An almost uncanny ability to be present in the moment, strong ability to hyperfocus on something interesting or important, and the capacity to see what others don't see.

**Cons:** Can appear selfish because the child only does what he "wants" to do.

## EFFORT MANAGEMENT

*Alertness, Sustaining Effort, Managing Energy, and Processing Speed*

**What it looks like:** Extreme fatigue (can hardly keep eyes open) when it's necessary to sit and be quiet, trouble maintaining alertness, requirement of steady stimulation or feedback (physical or mental) to stay alert, and slow processing speed (takes a long time to read and/or write); or if hyperactivity kicks in, a hard time slowing down enough to ensure quality work. Needs stimulation to get and stay engaged.

**Pros:** The need to consciously manage effort and alertness can lead to improved self-awareness and self-care. Slow processing speed allows individuals to slow down and think before acting.

**Cons:** Lack of effort can appear lazy, slow processing speed (taking longer to do seemingly simple tasks) is often interpreted as stupid, and overly energetic behavior may be seen as a bit crazy or too much to handle, and can cause kids to rush through their schoolwork.

## EMOTION MANAGEMENT

*Managing Frustration and Modulating Emotions*

**What it looks like:** Low threshold for frustration (short fuse), difficulty regulating emotions, oversensitivity, inappropriate responses, easily overwhelmed by emotions, and a high propensity for drama.

**Pros:** Tendency to be incredibly empathetic and often very attentive to friends. (Management of this challenge leads to significant improvements in self-awareness.)

**Cons:** Can appear too angry or too sensitive.

## INFORMATION MANAGEMENT (MEMORY)

*Using Working Memory and Accessing Recall*

**What it looks like:** Challenged in actively holding one piece of information in mind while working on another. Academically, for example, a child might have difficulty keeping track of a subtotal while performing an additional computation in a math problem. Or, in everyday life, a child might become distracted by something else when setting out to do a task (you might call this the "What did I come in here for?" phenomenon).

**Pros:** Tendency to forget allows people to repair relationships after fights and keeps them from holding a grudge. We've seen that people with ADHD often let go of minor upsets more easily than their friends and family members.

**Cons:** Can appear disobedient or sometimes stupid.

## ACTION MANAGEMENT

*Monitoring, Inhibiting, and Self-Regulating Action*

**What it looks like:** Hyperactivity and impulsivity, or when to act versus when to not act, such as assessing and determining when to tell a joke, confront a friend or family member, or speak in class or in a conversation. Distractibility and working memory challenges often make people behave in a more random manner than others, and impulsivity can cause frequent interruption.

**Pros:** If exercise is used to manage action, improved physical health can result. A tendency to say "yes" and take on new responsibilities can lead to opportunities for leadership development.

**Cons:** Can appear as being all over the place, clumsy, or even sometimes socially awkward. Tendency to overcommit can lead to stress and disappointment.

## Common Treatments for ADHD

Treatments for ADHD fall into two categories: medical and behavioral. Ideally, they work best when used together. In about 80 percent of people, some of the challenges of ADHD are improved by medication. But even if medication is effective, it does not address all of the challenges of ADHD. **Behavioral interventions are necessary for long-term success in managing the condition.** When children are involved, behavioral management starts with the parents.

### PARENT TRAINING/BEHAVIOR THERAPY

It may surprise you to learn that the most recommended treatment for young children (under age six) with ADHD is not medication—it's behavior therapy. Behavior therapy may be referred to as "behavior-management training for parents," "parent behavior therapy," "behavioral parent training," or just "parent training." According to the American Academy of Pediatrics, the recommended treatment for children ages 6 to 11 with ADHD is a combination of medication and behavioral parent training.

Behavioral parent training focuses on educating the adults in a child's life—usually parents and sometimes teachers. According to the CDC, behavioral parent training teaches adults "how to create structure and reinforce good behavior" in kids with ADHD. Because children with ADHD struggle with the ability to pay attention, and their disruptive behaviors often cause challenges in relationships, parent training teaches parents how "to learn or strengthen positive behaviors and eliminate unwanted or problem behaviors."

In the May 2016 ADDitude webinar "More Than Meds: A Parent's Guide to Using Behavioral Therapy," William Pelham Jr. said, "Teaching parenting skills is the single most effective and important intervention for treating kids with ADHD." He went on to say, "There's no therapy that a therapist can do in their office with a child who has ADHD that will have any impact on that child's behavior." According to Dr. Pelham, parent training using behavioral strategies "is the only therapy that works."

How can you encourage your kids to embrace meditation?

- **Start with yourself.** How did you teach your child to talk? By talking to her and with others while around her. It's the same with meditation: You teach by example. Many parents have their own practice. If not, consider cultivating one. Start small, and set aside five minutes to meditate, or try a meditative silent walk or a yoga class.
- **Let your kids see you practice.** When you have a meditation practice, let your kids see it and know about it. Let them know if you're going to a class or waking up early to meditate. And bring it into your daily life. If, for instance, you feel your stress level rising, say, "Wait a second, honey. I'm going to take a deep breath and calm down because I feel myself getting upset." Moments of meditation can be as simple as taking deep breaths or waiting a few seconds before responding to a situation. However you connect with meditation, make sure you share it clearly with your children.
- **Involve them.** Keep it simple. You could, for instance, sit quietly all together for five minutes in the morning. If bedtime is a struggle or your child has sleep difficulties, try setting aside time each evening for relaxing with soothing music. The great part is that, as your child grows, she can take these techniques and adapt them to her developmental level.

## Calm the Brain with Physical Activity

Hyperactive children with ADHD may feel like their brains are moving a thousand miles a minute. In the same way it can activate the brain of a child with attention problems (see "Get Moving" on page 46), movement can help children with hyperactivity think more clearly and process information more effectively.

Although allowing a hyperactive child to move regularly in the course of a normal day is quite helpful, encourage your child with ADHD to be active—have him join a sports team or arrange for time at the playground where he can climb the monkey bars, swing, slide, and run around. Remember, movement helps organize a child's thinking and can put an abundance of hyperactive energy to productive use; instead of trying to stop your child's constant need for movement, harness it—both on and off the playing field.

## Allow Your Child to Not Be Still

Whenever and wherever possible, allow your child to stand or move when the reverse would be generally expected. There are certainly some places where you cannot make that accommodation (in that case, see "Fidget to Focus" on page 67); but generally speaking if you take the pressure off of your child to be still all the time, you'll notice his behavior start to improve.

Try a swivel chair at the dinner table or allow your child to stand while eating. Get a large exercise ball or bouncy ball for him to sit on during homework time or allow your child to lie down during this time so he can bounce his feet or legs off the edge of a couch . . . or table (Elaine's daughter enjoys doing her homework while lying on the dining room table!). You can allow dancing in the seatbelt in the car or while setting the table for dinner. If the movement doesn't interfere, then let your child move.

Of course, there will be times when you need to still a bouncing knee that is distracting you from an important family conversation, but you can do that more easily and with less reaction from your child if you ease up on constantly trying to harness the energy of his sometimes racehorse-levels of movement.

## Give 'em a Job

Kids like to feel productive and helpful. Most kids want to follow directions and be seen as a good kid. But, sadly, kids with ADHD often feel bad, thinking they can't do anything right or they're always causing trouble. They don't mean to cause trouble, but that Energizer Bunny inside them is running on a perpetual battery.

One way to help your child productively channel his energy is to give him a job to do. Assign your child to be the "hopper" at dinnertime, and let him be the one to hop up to get the ketchup or the extra napkins for the table. Or make him the "master scrambled egg maker" or "strawberry de-stemmer." Enlist him to carry in the groceries and/or take the groceries out of the bags. Your child can be in charge of feeding your animals or watering the plants, too. Talk with your child about other ways to channel all that energy for productive use.

Ask your child's teacher if he or she can enlist your child's help passing out worksheets, collecting workbooks, and other tasks that allow some movement in the classroom. Speak with your child's sports coaches about giving your child a chance to play a position that involves movement, like the catcher in baseball, rather than standing around in the outfield picking flowers.

## Target Physical Activity Before and During Brainwork

Building on the previous strategies, use physical movement to heighten your child's ability to focus when she has a task to do that requires brainwork. Research has shown that kids who run around for 10 minutes before taking a test perform better than kids who have to sit still before taking the test. Help your child understand that movement is a strategy she can use to help her be successful. When there is homework to do or a book to read, or, for older kids, an application to fill out, pairing movement with brainwork can significantly improve the outcome.

Before your child begins an activity that requires brainwork, encourage 10 minutes of physically active play. The wheelbarrow game is a great activity for this. Have your child get on all fours, then carefully lift her legs and "wheel" her around the house for a few minutes to get her body engaged. Having her run around outside or at the playground is a good idea as well. Encourage your child to do a few push-ups or pull-ups on a chin-up bar before getting down to work. (A chin-up bar is a staple tool for managing ADHD for kids of all ages.)

Movement while studying can be helpful as well. For example, bounce and pass a ball back and forth with your child while reviewing vocabulary words, or suggest he bounce a ball while memorizing a poem. A trampoline, if you are so inclined, can be another great tool. Your child can bounce while studying math or telling you about the book he's reading. Chairs that bounce or seat cushions that wiggle are also useful when it's time to take a seat.

## Double-Tasking

Double-tasking (or attention switching) is a great ADHD strategy to help kids stay on task and complete projects. It's not multitasking, which is doing multiple things at once. Your brain cannot actually do two things simultaneously—even if you think it can! The ADHD brain is likely to get distracted or bored while performing a task. So instead of trying harder to stay focused on one task, plan something else constructive to do for when your child has lost interest in a task—that's double-tasking. This is a proactive solution for ADHD brains that get easily bored. The point is to keep your child engaged and interested by anticipating distraction and planning for it.

Here's how it works: Instead of assigning only one activity at a time (e.g., math homework), give your child *two* things to work on over a period of time (e.g., "In the next hour, you'll be working on math and watching a history video"). He begins with one task, but he knows that when he's ready to stop, he can switch to the other. With two projects going at once, he can move between them when he notices that his attention starts to wander or his enthusiasm wanes. Instead of setting aside the math and doing some other random activity, double-tasking sets the intention that when he gets bored (and he probably will), the other task is waiting.

Other examples of double-tasking include studying for a test for 10 minutes, then switching to vocabulary words for 10 minutes, and then back to the test for 10 minutes, and so on. This works for household tasks, too, like cleaning his room and doing laundry.

## Fidget to Focus

One terrific tactic to allow kids to move without disrupting others—while keeping their brain engaged—is through conscious fidgeting. Adults do this all the time. Classic examples of this strategy include chewing on a pencil or pen, twirling pieces of scrap paper in a meeting, or doodling in a notebook. Kids who need to fidget are often found biting their nails or even chewing on their hair or clothing.

When our kids (and their teachers) understand that fidgeting can be helpful, we can teach them to do it constructively. Some kids are allowed to chew gum in class as part of an Individualized Education Plan (IEP), because the chewing helps their brains stay engaged. Other strategies in the classroom include allowing the child to hold a small "fidget"—for instance, a smooth stone, squeeze ball, or small lump of modeling clay.

You can allow your child to bring a Rubik's Cube to a concert, for instance, or color quietly during religious services. Magnetic Buckyballs can keep a child occupied during long drives or while waiting at the doctor's office. Fidgets are also helpful while standing when larger movements are not an accommodation you can make.

You will need to set agreements with your child (and the teacher if the fidget is used in class) to make sure she doesn't hyperfocus on it, but generally speaking, when a child can keep her fingers engaged, it's easier for her to keep her brain engaged and helps her remain in one position. When you use this strategy, you'll find that not as much redirection is required, and your child begins to assume responsibility for managing her hyperactivity.

## Become a Scribe

Writing is one of the most complex tasks we ask kids to do. It involves almost every aspect of executive function, as well as a significant amount of motor coordination. When we expect kids to plan, prioritize, think critically, sequence, organize—*and* hold the pen and shape the letters, or type at the same time—their brains can wear out quickly.

Scribing (writing or typing for your child) is a terrific accommodation to support kids who struggle with planning and writing and a wide range of other school-related challenges, especially in the case of dysgraphia—a learning disability that affects the ability to write coherently. (One of our daughters has dysgraphia, and she likes it when Mom writes because it's neater and easier for her to read.) It also helps a child whose chief challenge is anxiety.

You would not use this strategy if the point of the assignment is handwriting. But for most schoolwork, providing motor support (scribing) can free up children's brains to do the real thinking that an assignment requires. It helps them get the thoughts out of their heads because they aren't getting stuck in the mechanics of writing. (One of our sons likes the writing support so he can think out loud and not have to write it down at the same time.)

For younger kids, being a scribe might involve writing down their vocabulary sentences as they recite them to you, or capturing a story they tell you. For older kids, it might involve taking notes while they think through their homework assignments or letting them dictate an essay to you.

When you are your child's scribe, put on your court reporter hat and avoid the tendency to correct or do the homework for your child. Your job as a scribe is to record your child's efforts so he can pay attention to the job of learning. It's okay to suggest a word or ask if he might want to express something in a different way, but for the most part, try to keep yourself out of the content of your child's work.

## Bring Activities Everywhere

This may seem obvious, but we want to be really clear: Kids who struggle with hyperactivity need a constant outlet for activity. They need to be doing something *all the time*, because their brains are constantly seeking stimulation.

Sure, sometimes it's great for kids to get bored and figure out how to entertain themselves to challenge their creativity, but there are times when you want them to be able to pay attention, wait patiently, or otherwise curb their enthusiasm when you're out and about in the world. In those cases, you can either give them something to do or find that they're doing something that may not be what you had in mind.

So, like a good Boy Scout, be prepared. For children under age 10, travel with books, sudoku puzzles, Rubik's Cubes, squeeze balls, crayons and coloring books, and scissors and paper. Fill a tote bag with whatever you know normally engages your child. As your child gets older, you can involve him in filling a small tote bag of items that will keep him busy during downtime.

Here's an important note: Try to disregard the judgmental stares of other parents whose children are sitting quietly with their hands in their laps while your child is coloring or snipping away. Your child is not wired to sit quietly with his hands in his lap, and there's really no great virtue in it anyway!

## Busy Boxes and Junk Boxes

Busy boxes and junk boxes (collections of busy-keeping items) recognize your child's busy brain and reward her for her creativity. They are particularly wonderful for helping children age 10 and younger manage attention, impulsivity, and hyperactivity. When you hear the inevitable "I'm bored" comment, direct your child to her busy box or junk box and see what she can come up with to entertain herself. Here are some ideas:

- **Busy box:** Set aside a large box or even shelf space in your home and fill it with toys your child can play with or activities that your child can do independently. Change out the toys and activities occasionally so there's always something new to discover. Have at least a few favorite items that live only in the busy box to keep those things novel.

- **Junk box:** One person's junk is another person's treasure. No one is better at discovering treasures than hyperactive kids with creative brains. Collect loose items, everyday household discards, and other objects you might call found art. An empty toilet paper roll, a plastic spiral binder from a discarded notebook, scraps of fabric, and leftover game pieces are all candidates for the junk box. Anything that's safe (nothing sharp) is fair game. These random items provide fuel for some of the most unusual art projects your child will ever create.

## Gamify Routine Tasks and Chores

The ADHD brain needs to be motivated to get things done. Two of the key avenues for motivation are play and competition. If you can make a game out of something—in other words, "gamify" it—it increases the likelihood of gaining and holding your child's attention, and the chance that he'll stick with the activity long enough to learn a new habit. Besides, games are the currency of the digital generation.

We do this naturally when our kids are little, but as they get older, we forget how effective it can be to march to the van for ballet or soccer, clean off the kitchen counters while singing Aretha at full volume into a wooden spoon, or race against the clock to see who can get up the stairs first to get ready for bed. Even the most boring dinner can become a special event if served on finger-food night—especially if you are brave enough to serve mashed potatoes. Take those superheroes (complete with cape and shorts over leggings) to the grocery store. See how fast you can unload the dishwasher before it's time to watch a family movie.

When you gamify chores, will there be times when things are done too fast and not quite as carefully as you might like? Sure. You might not want to make a game of folding shirts—that's complicated enough as it is! But there is a trade-off involved. If you're getting your child into the habit of unloading the dishwasher, you can trust that over time, he'll learn to dry off the silverware before putting it in the tray. If he's shooting hoops with his laundry, he can pick up the clothes that missed the hamper and try again with the chance to make a basket.

Not all games have to be competitive. Competition is a strong motivator for some kids, but it's the opposite for others. If your child does not have a good tolerance for the frustration of losing a game, or if your child is still extremely sensitive about doing *anything* wrong, focus on the play part of creating games without the emphasis on winners and losers.

## Flexible Homework Stations and Times

Warning: This strategy flies in the face of traditional recommendations. We hear from the experts all the time how important it is to be consistent. "Have your kids do their homework in the same place, at the same time," the experts tell us. Or, "Make sure they are sitting properly at a desk when doing their homework."

That may be true for neurotypical kids, and even for some kids with ADHD, but it can be a recipe for failure for many other kids with ADHD. Our kids are wired differently, and we need to understand and respect that. Doing homework in the same place every day can get boring really quickly. And honestly, most of our kids have been struggling to sit at a desk all day. They need a little freedom to move around. The same is true for expecting your child to do homework at the same time. Some days, it's just not going to be a good fit.

You can apply this strategy differently, depending on what's important to you. If you feel that some structure is important, you might want to set up a few different homework stations that your child can choose from each day, and two different options for when she might do her homework. Then, after school you can ask, "When are you planning to do your homework, and what station are you choosing tonight?" You may discover that if your child does not get her homework done by 5:00, it's best to plan to wake up a little early and have her do it in the morning, rather than waste hours trying to get 10 minutes of homework completed.

If you're willing to let your child do homework where she wants, then you don't need to have formal homework stations. In that case, you can ask, "Where do you feel like doing your homework tonight?" The kids in our families have done homework on the dining room table, under the kitchen table, and in a tree outside (family rule: only reading in the tree). The only condition here (besides safety) is that homework is done in a reasonable time frame. Before allowing this kind of freedom, set the expectation that you'll check in with each other to make sure it's working and agree to reconsider if it seems to be too distracting.

The key is to do a little detective work to figure out what works best for your kid (and for you) to provide her with some flexibility within the structure, along with some sense of control. You're holding her accountable to do her homework, but you're giving her some freedom to figure out when and where. That offers a strong sense of ownership and buy-in—which becomes critical as your child gets older and needs to be fully responsible for her schoolwork.

This strategy applies to older kids and teens, as well. Studying with friends at a local coffee shop may be a terrific option. As long as the work is getting done, letting your child decide how and when she completes her work fosters greater independence.

## The Personal Cave

Hyperactivity is one manifestation of your child's challenges with regulating energy—overstimulation is another. If your child is the one spinning around like the Tasmanian Devil, he's likely fine; but put him in a room with other chaotic energy—a loud television or music, a screaming or screeching sibling, or an angry parent—and he may become quite overwhelmed. So instead of waiting until your child shuts down, give him a space where he can go to recuperate—a personal cave.

This personal cave will allow your child to retreat or escape from the intensity of the environment long enough to center himself. It doesn't have to be a lot of space—just a designated space that is guaranteed to let your child be alone for a few minutes to regroup. It's like a restorative, self-imposed time-out space.

Where should you create this personal cave? One of our sons created a "man cave" for himself by draping an extra sheet over his L-shaped bunk beds. Other ideas include a good climbing tree, a pop-up tent, a spacious closet that's not full of junk, or even a window seat. It's most important that your child sees it as a safe, private space.

This is also an effective strategy for kids who struggle with emotional intensity and for any child who wants some private quiet time.

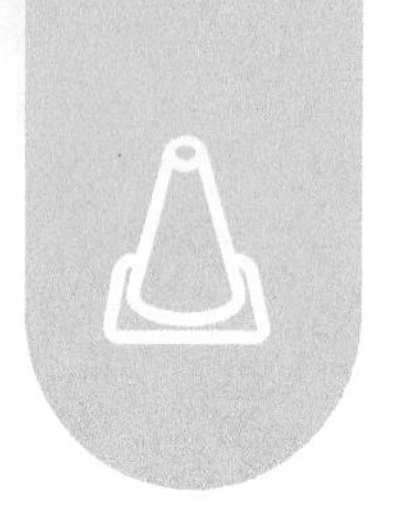

CHAPTER 5

# Curbing and Managing Impulsivity

In this chapter, you'll find tips, tricks, tactics, and strategies to address problems with managing impulsivity. The strategies outlined here are effective for a child who struggles with inhibiting impulses—which make it difficult to think before acting, follow directions, wait for a turn, and generally react or behave appropriately. Children who are excessively silly or overly aggressive often struggle with impulsivity and tend to be unaware of their impact on others.

The key executive function deficits that need to be addressed when managing challenges with impulsivity are:

- **Effort Management:** alertness, sustaining effort, managing energy, and processing speed
- **Emotion Management:** managing frustration and modulating emotions
- **Information Management (Memory):** using working memory and accessing recall
- **Action Management:** monitoring, inhibiting, and self-regulating action

## Positive Communication: Three Steps to Redirect

Impulsivity presents in many ways for our kids, so it can be incredibly difficult to manage. Impulsivity touches on at least four out of the six key aspects of executive function that are impacted by ADHD. It causes frustration for parents and kids alike and interferes with productivity and relationships.

As parents, staying positive can be difficult when your child seems to be out of control. To redirect your child, employ the ACE (acknowledge, compassion, explore options) steps. When you understand that your child is not being lazy, rude, or intentionally disrespectful, use ACE to help you respond to and redirect challenges with impulsivity (and other challenges of ADHD), and problem-solve to help your child learn self-regulation and self-management. Here are the steps:

1. **Acknowledge.** Name it. Acknowledge what's going on for your child so she can begin to recognize it herself. ("Wow, you were standing on the counter. I'm guessing you forgot that you're not supposed to do that, huh?" or "When your sister's backpack knocked into you, that must have really surprised you. I know you didn't want to hurt her, and that it was an instinct to hit back when you thought you were being hit.") When you start to acknowledge that your child is struggling with something, it will help your child not feel wrong but instead feel empowered to try to handle things differently in the future.
2. **Compassion.** Show your understanding. Have compassion for the mistake your child made so she can recognize what happened without feeling judged. ("It's hard for me to control myself, too, when I'm really excited about something," or "I get really freaked out when I get startled, too, and sometimes I can't control myself. It's like what happens when I see a cockroach, right?"). Humor is always an added bonus.



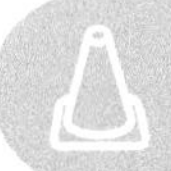

3. **Explore Options.** Work it out. Explore options for how to handle things differently in the future. Redirect the behavior or problem-solve as appropriate. Maybe you negotiate a compromise or create a code word (see page 88). Allow your child to regain a sense of control. For example, you might say, "When you're trying to reach something that's too high, I'd prefer if you ask for help. But maybe you're getting old enough to use a step stool, too. What do you think? How do you think you might remember not to climb up on the counters?" or "We might want to come up with some strategies to use when you get startled so you don't lash out and hurt people unintentionally. Would you like that? I know you love your sister and didn't mean to hurt her. Why don't we make sure she's okay and apologize to her first, and then we can come up with some other strategies for the future when you're ready. What do you think about that plan?"

## Setting Realistic Expectations: Remind Without Nagging

One of the most common questions we hear from parents in coaching sessions and on training calls is "How do I say it in a way that my child will respond?" How do you give your kids directions without triggering a reaction? How do you get them to do their homework without starting a fight? How do you remind them to do what you've asked without sounding like a nag? You know the challenges—the list could go on.

Applying ACE goes a long way toward helping you communicate with your kids—it fosters connection and cultivates independence. But sometimes you also have to break some old habits—yours, not theirs. It is every bit as important to pay attention to *how* you're speaking to your kids as it is to what you actually say.

More than likely, when you generate negative responses from your kids, there are two things going on. First, kids with ADHD often hear neutral comments as criticism because they are hypersensitive to negative feedback. Second, there may well be

an underlying message that you are not saying directly but they are hearing loud and clear, like "You messed up again" or "I feel like I can't count on you." Even when our intentions are good, we say things in a way that sounds judgmental or accidentally puts our kids on the defensive. We don't mean for that to happen, of course—but we *all* do it. So when your child responds negatively, you may get triggered in return . . . and a vicious cycle continues.

Changing your tone starts with shifting your expectations and becoming aware of the unintended messages you are actually sending—so that you can choose the messages you want to send. For example, consider classic parent statements like "Why can't you just . . . ?" "Why don't you ever remember to . . . ?" "When are you going to . . . ?" and the most famous one of all, "How many times do I have to tell you?"

Now, take a moment to think about the messages behind those questions. What are we really saying when we ask most of these questions? Usually, the unspoken message is some variation of "You're failing," or—worse for your child than that—"You're a failure." It's not exactly a strong motivator for your child to get up and do what you've asked.

So start by shifting your own expectations. Remember, there is a good reason why he can't just . . . why he doesn't remember to . . . why he hasn't yet. . . . And most of all, remember that *you are very likely going to need to repeat yourself.* That is a fundamental truth of parenting, even with kids who don't have ADHD. It is all the more likely for kids with ADHD who struggle with attention, working memory issues, and all the other challenges of executive function.

Expect that your child is going to need reminders and redirection. That is our job as parents. When we take away the nagging nature of the communication by making it routine, we are freed to help our kids learn, instead of judging them for what they have not yet mastered. Instead of asking, "How many times do I have to tell you?" you might say, "It seems like you might need a reminder about this. How would you like me to remind you? And how many times do you think is reasonable?" Remember that your child may not know, but it can be a great place to do some detective work together!



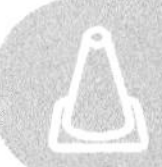

If you understand and expect that your child is going to need reminders, then you won't be disappointed when it happens. And you'll be in a much stronger position to pass the baton to your child over time. When you make reminders routine, your child will be more willing to set up reminders for herself as she matures and takes on new levels of responsibility.

## The Power of the Pause

Never underestimate the value of taking a break, a pause, or a breather, whether it's deep breathing, counting to 10, or walking away before reacting. Most of us know that hitting pause during stressful, emotional, or intense moments has the power to diffuse even the most difficult situations, even though it can be really hard to do. While pausing helps with managing every challenging aspect of ADHD, it is particularly helpful for curbing impulsivity.

Children who struggle with impulsivity tend to be managed by the moment and often have a limited tolerance for frustration, difficulty coping with intense emotions, and lag behind their peers in some aspects of maturity. They are not likely to learn self-control automatically—they need to be taught. And one key way to do that is by teaching them to consciously slow down and notice—anything and everything.

Kids with impulsivity need to know when to act and when not to. To develop that awareness, they need to learn to regularly stop and think things through. Classic ADHD impulsivity happens because action comes before thinking. Pausing shifts that dynamic. This is a two-step process:

1. Practice pausing—often.
2. Verbalize what you're doing and let it help you communicate clear expectations.

How do you practice pausing? Stop before doing something, such as before getting out of the car to go into the grocery store. Help your child think through what to expect inside the store. Articulate what challenges your child might face in a bright store with lots of distractions (and candy!), and verbalize the behaviors you would

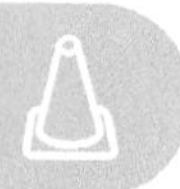

like to encourage. Then, before you leave the store, pause a moment to look around. Verbalize that you want to make sure you have all your belongings and that you have everything you went in for. You can do this before any activity or anyplace you visit.

Pauses don't always have to be productive. You can pause to take a deep breath, to smile at your child and give a hug, or even to just take a moment before moving on to what's next. When you take the time to pause and verbalize it, you're teaching your child a lifelong skill for self-regulation and self-management.

## Deep, Calming Breaths

Like pausing, deep, calming breaths can restore calm, redirect negativity, and ease impulsivity. Taking deep, calming breaths can reverse some of our fight-or-flight response by counteracting the production of stress hormones and reducing our heart rate and blood pressure. The next time you feel your pulse racing, follow these steps:

1. Stop whatever you are doing.
2. Take three to five slow, deep breaths. As you do so, focus on making your exhale longer than your inhale (this relaxes the body).
3. Ask yourself, "How do I want to respond?"
4. If you breathe before reacting, there is a good chance that you will change your response and avoid those "Why did I say that?" situations.

Teach your child the importance of deep, calming breaths, too, and practice with him. With this tool on hand, your child can learn to diffuse intense moments at home, at school, and when playing with friends.

## Make a Game of Slowing Down

These days, we tend to move through life at a rapid pace. We make games of seeing how fast we can do something, and we are constantly urging our kids to hurry up! Sometimes, that is a terrific



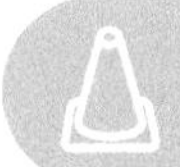

strategy to help us get it all done. But there is also a value in slowing things down—especially for kids under age 10 who tend to act without thinking. We often talk about it in terms of slowing down to speed up (see page 130 for more on this).

This strategy reinforces and builds on the power of the pause, taking it a step further. It is about practicing the process of slowing things down in all different aspects of life. There are several ways to make a game out of slowing things down. Start talking in slow motion, and encourage your kid to join you. Or see how slowly you can pour milk into the cereal or chew a bite of dinner. This is really a technique from mindfulness (see page 61), and it can do a lot to raise awareness of how fast we tend to go, and how hard it is to pay attention or control our actions when we're moving so fast.

A really fun way to teach this to your kids is to have them walk (not run) as quickly as they can around the house (you can also do this outside). Tell them to keep going for a while, and notice what they can pay attention to around them when they're moving really fast. Then ask them to cut it to half speed and tell you what they are able to notice. Do that for a while, and then cut it to half speed again. Do this several times until they are barely moving and are talking in slow motion. Not only can it be a lot of fun, but it also helps them see that there is a lot of stuff they are missing when they are racing through life. Not that racing is bad—sometimes it's exhilarating. But we want to teach them the value in slowing down, too.

## Brain Breaks

"All work and no play makes Jack a dull boy." In fact—Jack's brain can't really work effectively if it's always in overdrive. Have you ever been in a situation where your kid took three hours to do 10 minutes of homework? Our tendency is to try to push them through the work, to focus on getting it done. But what they might really need more than that is to *stop*. Brain breaks help kids slow things down and self-manage, which are critical to curbing impulsivity.

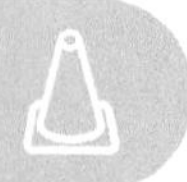

Although the ADHD brain seems to run a million miles an hour, it gets easily fatigued (probably because it's running a million miles an hour!). Frequent breaks are a must to refresh and reengage—and avoid the boredom that comes from working on the same thing for hours. Even if your kid isn't struggling, frequent breaks can keep things moving forward at a steady pace and be a good practice for brain health.

Your child can do some jumping jacks, have a tickle fight, eat a snack, or sing a song. Maybe he can read the comics after finishing his math, or if you think your child can do it without getting sucked in, he can watch a silly three-minute YouTube video. Keep the brain fresh and engaged so it can more easily get the work done. By the way, this tip will work for you as well, whether your challenge is an ADHD brain, or just a tired, worn-out parent!

## Say Yes More Often

It's amazing how often we say the word *no*. Kids with ADHD probably hear it more often than most, because they are frequently doing something out of line. In intimate relationships, the ideal is to give five positive comments to every negative one—but it's not so easy to do!

Whenever reasonable, try to agree to your child's requests and say yes. This doesn't mean you never say no, but it does mean that you consider "How can I make this a yes?" It also means that when you do say no, you provide the child with a reason, even if that reason is "I'm sorry, but I'm too tired and tonight isn't a convenient night for me."

If you think about it, we often say "no" more than necessary, and this prevents a terrific opportunity to foster independence. When you really look at why you're saying no, oftentimes you can turn it into a chance to teach a little responsibility. For example:

- Child asks, "Can I clean up my bedroom *after* I watch my show?"
- Parent thinks about it, and then says, "As long as your room is done by 1 p.m., when we need to leave for our appointment, I don't mind. What is your plan for getting it done by then?"



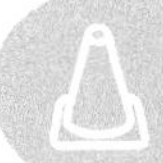

While the goal in saying yes more often is to be a more positive and supportive parent, it comes with a few added bonuses:

- Your kids will trust you more. They know that you are on their side, and when you do have to turn down a request, they may be more willing to trust that your reasons are justified and you are not just pulling rank on them as a parent.
- Saying positive things supports not only your kid but you as well. It feels good to say yes and give positive feedback.

Don't feel like you have to get out a counter and keep track of the 5:1 ratio, but do make an effort to yes more often. Before you say no, make sure you understand why you are saying it, and see if you might be able to find a way to turn it into a yes.

## Celebrate Being Good

Building on the "Say Yes More Often" strategy (on page 81), we can shift that 5:1 ratio to more positive statements by catching our kids being good. Think about it: We catch them being "bad" all the time. Sometimes, we even look for the mistakes. But celebrating the good stuff—and helping them see when they are doing it—is a great way to enhance their self-awareness, which leads to self-control.

Celebration is the act of honoring a person or event. In families, this is easy to do when it's a defined event: birthdays, report cards, holidays, and so on. But we can also celebrate daily behaviors, like being nice to your sister, following directions, or helping a friend. In our community, one family celebrated staying in church one to five minutes longer each week. It took a full year to be able to make it through a one-hour service (even with a busy bag and snacks), but celebrating each step along the way kept their son with ADHD focused on the successes and motivated all year! Celebrating with our kids makes them feel good about themselves, and it can be a powerful motivator.

So celebrate their successes—both the big and small! Notice their accomplishments. Catch them being good. Find things to brag about to your friends and family members. Every day, find

something in your children's lives to honor. In truth, you'll most likely enjoy it more than they will. Success breeds success, so jump up and down and do a happy dance when the achievements happen—and make sure your kid learns to celebrate his success, too!

## Token Economy

One of the most common ADHD strategies is the token economy, otherwise known as a reward system. Because our kids do not yet have the internal controls to help them remember what they should or shouldn't do and when, rewards (such as stickers, stars, or whatever symbols or incentives you decide to use) provide external support. For a child with ADHD, rewards or incentives can make the difference between negative behaviors that strain relationships and positive behaviors that lead to happier, healthier families.

Why not consequences? Threats, yelling, or taking away privileges can send kids with ADHD into panic mode and make it difficult for them to access the problem-solving portion of their brains. Besides creating stress, the immediate results don't last. They don't learn a lesson when you threaten to take away the tablet or video game. They respond out of fear or anxiety.

Rewards work quite well for our kids because they are based on motivation, not punishment. Rewards recognize positive behaviors and encourage more of them. They focus on what your kid is doing right, rather than what she's doing wrong.

Behavior management systems like a token economy can be hard to maintain! Parents who struggle with organization can find a token economy to be overwhelming—just one more thing to try to manage. So how can you make sure the system you put into place is effective and manageable? Follow these three simple steps:

1. **Identify *one* behavior you want to change.** Maybe it's your kid's inability to get ready for school and to the bus stop on time. Maybe it's the struggle at bedtime. Maybe it's the constant sassing. Maybe it's a million other things—*but pick only one*! Once you have a handle on that behavior, you can move on to



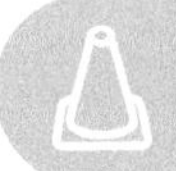

others. To keep your kid—and yourself—from becoming overwhelmed or defeated, focus on one behavior at a time.

2. **Identify your child's motivators.** The ADHD brain will not do anything unless it is genuinely interested or motivated. So what's the carrot that's going to motivate your kid? Is it an extra half-hour of screen time when she makes it to the bus on time? Is it an extra 15 minutes of story time before bed when she puts away her toys? Or a chance to have a favorite dessert when she earns three stickers (or checkmarks) for talking respectfully at dinnertime?
3. **Start a feedback loop.** In your system, make sure that you have a way to measure progress or determine whether your child is engaging in the desired behavior. If, for instance, you want her to brush her teeth every night, how are you going to ensure she does it? And when she starts to do it consistently, what's the next step? How can you move forward with this behavior? Maybe you move from doing it for her, to watching her. Finally, you send her up to do it herself, confident that she can and will. (Yes, you might test the toothbrush at first to see if it's wet, but she doesn't have to know that!)

Life is complicated enough. Reward systems work best when they're simple. So, what behavior do you want to change? What's going to make her want to change? And how are you going to know if she is making the change? That's it, in a nutshell. It doesn't have to—and shouldn't—be more complex than that.

A thoughtfully structured reward system is one of the most powerful tools in a parent's toolbox for behavior management. You can empower your child to make great changes, one step at a time, with an effective reward system. And as an added bonus, you'll go from feeling like the bad guy all the time to feeling like the superstar parent you are!

Success breeds success, and even if your child's wins are small, they count. Make sure she knows that! Rewards are a great way to show her, and yourself, that she's making progress, that you're doing something that's making a difference.

## Hand on the Arm

This is a strategy to support kids who struggle with interrupting, specifically kids who interrupt because they have a hard time managing impatience and get stuck in an "I need it now" mind-set.

Let's say you're on the phone. Your kid might be in the background trying to get your attention. "Mom, Mom, Mom . . . " He needs your attention right then! And he can't (yet) regulate his actions effectively to allow you to finish your conversation and then turn your focus to him. This strategy works like a charm for ages four and up to manage impulsive interruptions. It even works with teenagers!

1. When your child approaches and wants to say something, teach him to put his hand on your arm to get your attention.
2. Put your hand on his hand to acknowledge him. This signals to him that you understand he wants your attention, and you will get to him soon. No words are spoken, and your child has successfully avoided interrupting rudely. (You can celebrate that later!)
3. Find the quickest stopping point in your conversation to say "Excuse me" to whomever you're talking with, and turn your attention to your child—briefly! Giving quick access to you, so he knows you'll get to him, will help your child wait more patiently.
4. Unless it's *really* quick, don't engage whatever your child wants yet; just listen to a quick summary of what he wants to tell you. (It's okay to remind him to bottom-line it or make it quick.)
5. After you hear what he wants, ask him to wait a moment. Turn back to your original activity; continue talking or whatever you were doing. Now your child knows that he has your attention and you're going to get to him in a minute. This helps him practice waiting.
6. Again, as soon as you can comfortably do it, turn your attention back to your child. This time, either address the issue or set up a clear time when you will be available to address his



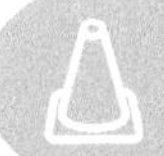

need or concern. (For example, if you can't address it right away, tell him you will talk about it or he can tell you all about it tonight during dinner. It's important to remember to come back to it!)

If this seems complicated, the key ideas are:

- Anticipate that interruptions are going to happen.
- Agree in advance on a way to handle them together.
- Show your child you intend to be attentive to his needs (putting your hand on his).
- Teach your child to wait patiently by gradually increasing the time he waits.

## Coffee-Filter Wisdom

Impulsivity and other challenges related to self-regulation can make life with ADHD chaotic. Often, kids (and adults) feel bewildered, as if they're navigating a world without a map that everyone else is using. This can lead to inappropriate behavior, acting out, and meltdowns.

This strategy is great for kids who get in trouble (with teachers or friends) for impulsively saying hurtful things. A client of ours came up with this idea after listening to one of our classes on impulsivity and emotionality. We thought it was so brilliant, we asked if we could share it with other parents. It helps you teach your child to consciously self-regulate, instead of being disappointed because it's so difficult for your child to manage his impulsivity and emotionality.

Here's how it works: Show your child a coffee filter and explain how it works. Explain that it holds the coffee in place and slows the water down so it has the time to seep through, collecting the flavor from the coffee. As an added bonus, it captures the bitter, gritty grinds so that delicious coffee is all that pours into the cup.

Then explain that when kids with ADHD struggle with impulsivity and emotionality, it's like they are missing the filter they need to slow their brains down and sort out the gritty grinds from their

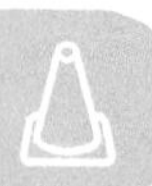

## CLARIFYING IMPULSIVITY

Of all the ways impulsivity presents in children with ADHD, perhaps the most common—and one of the most frustrating for teachers, parents, and peers—is interrupting. It happens at home and at school. Without a well-developed process for thinking through his actions, a child thinks of something and feels the need to express it immediately—before he forgets. Sometimes it comes from enthusiasm (he wants to participate in the class discussion or the conversation at the dinner table). Sometimes it comes from impatience (he can't wait for someone to finish a thought because he is so eager to share). Whatever is behind the interruption (wanting something now, wanting a parent to understand, wanting the teacher to know that he knows the answer), the child with ADHD has not yet developed the capacity to wait.

caring, loving thoughts. Without a filter, they often say things that they don't mean to say—things that can be hurtful to people they love. They say things they regret later.

Explain to your child that you understand that she struggles with this, and that you want to help her learn to filter her thoughts so that she will get better at thinking before she speaks. For starters, she can put the coffee filter in her pocket every day and just think about it throughout the day whenever she feels the filter. Then, if she gets frustrated, hurt, or angry, she can put her hand in her pocket and feel the coffee filter. It will remind her to take a few breaths or slow down before she says anything she might regret—or maybe not say anything at all until she's had a chance to think about it. Over time, explain that she will learn to filter her thoughts.

Remind her to be patient with herself because change takes time. Teach her to become aware of her reactions, because that is how she will learn to self-manage. When you treat mistakes as an opportunity for learning, you'll help your kid believe that she can do better, and not see herself as a bad kid.



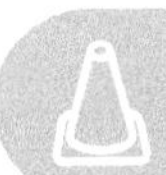

## Code Words

Code words are cues for redirecting behavior, words that family members or teachers agree upon to communicate a message quickly and without embarrassment. Code words help you get to the heart of a matter quickly, sort of like communicating in shorthand. The most commonly used code word most of us already know is "uncle." You call out "uncle" when you've had enough—when it's time to put a stop to something. It's a safe word, and most people know it means that a limit is being set. For the most part, it doesn't come with a lot of judgment or shame. It's a code word we all tend to accept and respect.

In our families, we use code words for all kinds of scenarios—to stop things before they escalate out of control, facilitate communication, ease emotionally intense situations, and aid in organization. Here are some code words Elaine's family uses:

- "Broccoli ice cream" is the code word for "someone is losing the ability to cope because he or she is hungry. Stop everything, now, and get some food!" (Elaine's family still uses it after more than 10 years.) Because the brain needs food for anything else to make sense, they focus there first.
- Someone was always getting hurt when her kids wrestled, but Elaine and her husband didn't want to stop all wrestling because they knew it was fun bonding for their kids. So a code word set the stage for the wrestling to happen with an agreed-upon limit in place. Her kids chose *basta* (which means "enough" in Spanish).
- "Rope" (as in "I'm at the end of my") means "Okay, everyone, back off because I'm trying really hard not to lose my cool."
- "Don't poke the bear" means "Leave your sister or brother alone because she's really not in the mood right now to be messed with."
- "Bubble gum" means "Brace yourself, because you might not like what I'm about to tell you, but I've still got to tell you, okay?"

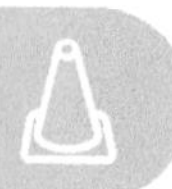

The key to success in using code words is agreement on the behavior you are trying to modify. You can't impose code words—they are best when they are a family creation. In fact, they don't often mean anything to anyone else, so they become a great inside joke for family bonding, as well. Here are some tips for developing code words:

- Figure out some behaviors that tend to cause problems repeatedly, and choose one area in which to start. (Note: Start simply with something your child wants to change, too. Get a win under your belt before moving to something more volatile.)
- Have a conversation about the idea of code words, and come to agreement that you want to give it a try. Let your child come up with the code word—and don't worry if it's ridiculous.
- Practice it a little bit by doing a role-play. Have some fun with it.
- Agree on the time frame in which you're going to try it before you check back in with each other—three days? one week? Whatever you agree upon is fine.
- Tweak and change, if necessary. You might need to change the word, or change the tone in which it's used, or even change the timing ("Don't ever use that when I'm in the bath, Mom—that's the one time it won't work for me"). Let your child have some ownership and help you fail forward by learning from what does and doesn't work.

The bottom line is that there are triggers in your family that could be avoided with a few well-chosen code words. If you're not sure, ask your kids. Not only will they probably know, but they'll also likely do a better job of naming them than you. After all—would *you* ever have come up with broccoli ice cream?



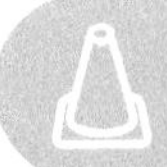

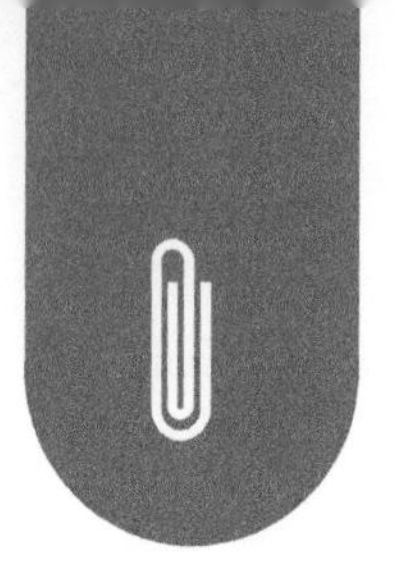

CHAPTER 6

# Getting Organized

In this chapter, you'll find tips, tricks, tactics, and strategies to address challenges with organization. These strategies are effective for a child who struggles with keeping track of belongings, following through on what is expected, and coping with a wide range of academic problems.

The key executive function deficits that need to be addressed when managing challenges with organization are:

- **Task Management (Activation):** prioritizing, organizing, and initiating activity
- **Attention Management (Focus):** focusing, sustaining, and shifting attention to tasks
- **Effort Management:** alertness, sustaining effort, managing energy, and processing speed
- **Information Management (Memory):** using working memory and accessing recall

## Positive Communication: Get Buy-In

As you know, finding motivation for anything and everything that needs to get done is critical for people with ADHD. Without motivation, many complex children lack the "just get it done" button in their brains that is required to activate and complete a task. Some motivators are external, like rewards. Other motivators are internal, like a sense of pride.

Buy-in—your child's willingness and desire to try a strategy—is a great way to cultivate a child's internal motivators. Buy-in offers a deeper commitment beyond surface rewards. Without buy-in, our kids may not have a stake in a task or an interest in finding the motivation to do it. But if they own the jobs, they're more likely to want to do them (or do them well) than if they think they're someone else's responsibility. External motivators can help kids get things done, but internal motivators will help them do those things again and again.

So what does this mean in practice? Your child has to understand and see value in any system or structure you are asking her to use. Is it reasonable? Does she believe she can do it? Does she *want* to do it? Does she believe it's going to work? What is her connection with the end result? What's important about it for her?

Before you try to put a new strategy in place, ask yourself, "What's in it for my child?" And then, bring your child into the process. If you want your child to get his homework done more efficiently, let him identify how it would benefit him. Let him get a sense of the value to him, rather than just feeling that he's doing it because you want him to do it. As you begin to shift ownership from you to him, the ideas become his, not yours.

Of course, this doesn't happen overnight—it takes time and patience to slowly pass the baton of ownership from you to your child. At first, there will likely be many things he still sees as something you are insisting that he needs to do. In those instances, focus on helping him find his own motivation for doing them, until your child begins to buy in to taking on new responsibilities as part of his own agenda.

A key element to getting a buy-in is making sure you're allowing your child to have a real say in developing any strategy. Make sure it works for him and is not just designed for how you would do it. For example, you may want your son to do his homework right after school at the kitchen table. But he might want to take a break, have a protein snack, do some pull-ups, and then do his homework at the dining room table or on the kitchen floor. What's most important is that he sees homework as his responsibility—something he's doing because he wants to do well in school, he wants to please his teachers, or whatever his reasoning may be. When he gets some say in *how* to do it, it increases a sense that it is his responsibility. It enhances his ownership. And that is the core of internal motivation.

## Setting Realistic Expectations: Focus on the Process

Our focus as a society seems to be on where we are going and not how we get there: "The ends justify the means." "Outcomes measurement." "Getting to the finish line." With kids with ADHD, this mind-set can lead to feelings of frustration and defeat, because the finish line often seems out of reach. So what should you focus on, if not the prize?

A key concept in managing executive function challenges is to hold your child (or yourself) accountable to the process rather than to outcomes. You want to reward your kid for using strategies rather than focusing too much on the strategy itself. This notion removes some pressure so kids can learn *how* to get the results they want.

Focusing on the process is a particularly important tool to foster long-term independence. We want our kids to begin to understand that it's going to be up to them to manage the details of their lives. Success with schoolwork is half cognitive and half organizational. So we want them to see that the process really *does* matter. It's like getting partial credit on a complicated math problem. *How* they do it is as important as it is for them to get the right answer.

For example, rather than focusing on finishing homework, you could hold your child accountable for staying on task for 10 to 20 minutes (depending on age and ability). Celebrate a success with a quick energy break or reward. If you stack a handful of these together, the homework can get done, typically with less stress. If your child is working on managing her emotions, you can base success on whether she uses self-calming strategies to calm down. Acknowledging the success is much more effective than punishing outbursts.

This is a helpful strategy to bring to conversations with the school, as well. Make sure reward systems in the classroom are focused on the process, not just on the results. Help teachers understand that learning *how* to learn, or calm down, or not blurt out in class is as important for your child as whether she masters this week's spelling words or does a five-page report. Focus on incremental steps of the process (one paragraph, instead of one page)—and allow your child to experience success along the way.

Success breeds success, so take the time to reward the use of strategies. It leads to improvement and increased self-esteem.

## Reassess Your Reward Strategy

Having a reward system in place to help your child get organized is a terrific strategy, as described in "Token Economy" on page 83. But despite your efforts, you might be disappointed that your kid hasn't reached for the rewards. It's possible your child might not be working for rewards because she is in some way scared, terrified, afraid of failure, or even afraid of her own success. (Yes, fear of success is very real! "If I do that well, then Mom will expect more from me!")

A lot of our kids struggle with anxiety—whether it's a coexisting diagnosis or the resulting frustration from the challenges of managing their ADHD. When anxiety rears its ugly head, it's extra hard to get *anything* done! When you're reassessing your reward system, be very clear on what you are rewarding. Is it a specific outcome? Or is it possibly just a reward for trying something, regardless of the results? That's a great way to use rewards when anxiety is clouding the picture. Did you include your child in the conversation, as discussed at the beginning of this chapter? Did she buy-in to the goal you've set? Are you on the same page with each other?

Make sure you are avoiding some of the common pitfalls with rewards:

- Not immediate enough—don't wait until the end of the day, week, or month when something can be rewarded more quickly. Particularly for younger children, make sure that rewards are given as soon as possible after the desired behavior.

- Rewards for multiple things at once—don't let rewards get so complicated that they are hard for you to deliver or difficult for your children to remember. It's best when it's simple and clear. When possible, try to work on only one, or up to three, behavior changes at a time.
- Notice if your child starts to feel defeated or gives up trying. It may be that the expectations are unrealistic. No matter how much a child wants a reward, if she doesn't think she can do what's asked of her, at some point she is likely to just stop trying.
- Canceling a reward that your child has earned because of a meltdown or other challenging behavior later in the day. If you child has earned the reward, you need to uphold your end of the deal.

## Keep Things Visual

Because of challenges with working memory and attention, some people with ADHD tend to organize themselves by field of vision. That is to say, if they can see it, they can remember it. Or the other way to look at it is "out of sight, out of mind." This explains why surfaces tend to be cluttered and things are often not put away—because as soon as a thing is put away, someone with ADHD might forget where he put it or forget that he ever even had it! It also contributes to time blindness, or the classic ADHD difficulty of keeping track of time.

The strategy here is to keep things more out in the open, where they are visible, than you might otherwise. We don't mean to keep it messy—it's best for everything to have a place. But the more people can see things, the better. Use cubbies or shelves instead of closed drawers; hang backpacks on a hook instead of closed in a closet; leave a child's morning checklist at her place at the table so she can see it instead of taped inside a kitchen cabinet. You might even keep medicine containers on the kitchen counter.

We understand that this is not a favorite strategy for highly organized people who like everything neatly tucked away behind closet doors, but it can make a world of difference for some people's ability to pay attention to what's important. So finding ways to keep things visually available, but still neat, will be a compromise well worth it for family peace.

Not *all* people with ADHD are visual, so you want to get a sense of whether your child tends to experience the world visually before incorporating this strategy into your lifestyle.

## Watch Time Pass

The challenges of time management can be incredibly stressful for parents. To address time-management challenges, choose strategies that bring attention to the passing of time. Visual timers, stop watches, and analog clocks help kids with ADHD get a handle on how long it takes to get things done and how things relate to each other in terms of time. We want them to *see* that time passes, not just think of it as an abstract concept.

Analog clocks and watches, in particular, are essential. Instead of seeing time as 10:45 on a digital clock, kids who learn to read an analog clock (or watch) understand that 10:45 is 15 minutes before the hour, thus reinforcing the passage of time. Some kids resist this because digital clocks are easier to read. But over time, we want to encourage them to process the information that time is not static, as seen on a digital clock face—it is constantly changing. This can be a great tool as well for kids who have issues with transitions.

## Prepare for Transitions

Attention challenges can be particularly difficult during times of transition, when kids are expected to stop focusing on one thing and turn their attention to another. This may be great for them if you're asking them to stop doing homework to join the family for movie night. But when the TV has to go off in order to get ready for bed, well, that can cause as much stress as Armageddon!

Remember that sometimes this applies even when you're asking your child to stop something he *doesn't* like, such as homework.

Even if he doesn't like it, he may want to please his teacher, you, or even himself—and he can start feeling stress if he's afraid he won't be able to do a good job. We all know that it's not likely that his "teacher is going to be so mad," but if he is genuinely concerned about that, it can be hard to get him to stop doing homework and go to bed on time.

You can't avoid transitions, but you can plan for them to reduce stress and teach your child to learn to handle frustration and disappointment. The following are a few tactics that can help for kids of different ages when they are struggling with stopping any kind of activity.

- **Give reminders.** Most kids do not have a strong sense of time, and this is especially true for children with ADHD. To set yourself and your child up for success, come to an agreement with each other about how much warning you'll give before he needs to stop a desired task. You might also agree on the number of warnings you'll give. One of our sons likes a 15-minute warning before dinner, and another one needs three reminders to get off of the computer.
- **Set timers.** As your children get older, you'll want to start gradually transferring the responsibility of reminders to them. You can teach a 6-year-old to use a timer, and a 10-year-old to use an alarm clock. Begin to hold them accountable to actually using the system they agree to use. For example, one of our sons is supposed to feed the dogs at 6:30, and his phone starts barking at him at 6:25. You can also use timers at regular intervals for kids to check in with themselves about how they're managing time. A timer that goes off every 10 or 20 minutes during homework time will help them to gauge how long it's taking them to get the work done, and remind them to get back on task if they've gotten distracted or to transition to the next assignment.
- **Require breaks during any long play.** One of the biggest challenges for parents is helping their child transition when she gets hyperfocused on something (remember the tip "Get Attention Before Giving Direction" on page 56). Because

regular brain breaks are really good for everyone, set the expectation that your child take breaks during elective activities, too—like playing video games. This is a great habit for kids to get into. Not only does it reinforce the importance of taking breaks, but it also gives their brains practice in stopping something once they're hyperfocusing. The process the brain needs to use to put on the brakes to stop playing a video game is not that different from the one to put down the pencil at the end of a standardized test. Besides, the more they learn to stop and start something really compelling to them, the better they'll be able to handle other transitions.

## Get Ready to Get Ready to Go

Most of us are living fast-paced lives, and we bounce from one activity to the next without a lot of time to prepare or breathe. While plenty of activity and engagement can be good for our kids, they also need time to slow down and plan—especially because it often doesn't come naturally to them.

Teach your child to plan enough time to transition from one thing to the next. You don't set your alarm in the morning for the time you want to leave the house; you set it early enough to get ready to leave the house. And this strategy should be encouraged for all the different activities of life. We need to build in an awareness of the time it takes to get ready to do anything. Before sitting down to dinner, maybe your child needs to build in an extra 20 minutes to feed the dogs, wash his hands, and set the table. He will need to stop whatever he is doing 20 minutes before dinner. Before going to sports practice, help him build in enough time for a snack and to put away some toys or do some homework.

When you're planning activities, show your child how you plan for transition time. Don't jump from one thing to the next without allowing a little wiggle room. When you know you're going to be leaving to go out to dinner, stop working or watching TV, or whatever is holding your attention, for long enough to get ready, find your phone and your keys, and figure out if you're going to need a jacket. This strategy, from coach Rudy Rodriguez can reduce stress in a lot of ways and model a terrific strategy for long-term time management.

## Homework Planning Process

Homework is hard for many kids with ADHD. Not only is it exhausting to have to go back to work after a long day at school, but quite often it's a challenge just to figure out what is expected of them. Even for little kids, there are so many different pieces to getting homework done. Then, as kids get older, there are multiple assignments by multiple teachers with staggering deadlines. It's an organizational feat just to know what work needs to be done each day.

Starting when she's young, teach your child to take the time to plan out homework. Not only will it help reduce overwhelming feelings, but it is a terrific way to teach lifelong planning skills. You'll want to offer to be a scribe (see page 67) for your child in this strategy, and it's okay to do that all the way through high school, if necessary. But if your child wants to write herself, definitely let her do it on her own. It won't be as neat as if you were to do it, but it will be hers, and that will enhance her buy-in. At some point, she will have to write on her own, of course, but when we can reduce that stressor, it allows her to focus on enhancing her thinking and planning.

Before you start, get buy-in to the process (see page 90). Ask your child if she's open to starting something new with you to help things go more smoothly and give her more time to play or do whatever else it is she wants to do. Let her choose a notebook to use regularly for homework planning (not too small), and explain that you're going to start on a new page every day. Here's the process:

1. **Capture Assignments**

   List each class or subject in school. Allow a few lines for each class/subject to capture multiple assignments.

Write down each task for each class that is due the *next* day. Your child might need to check an online portal or with a friend. Be patient while she figures out what is expected in each subject or class.

Ask if there are any ongoing projects that need to be considered. If it's a light homework day, that might be a good time to make some headway on a research paper. If it's a heavy-load day, or you know that your child will be short on time for another reason, you can leave this step out.

2 **Estimate Time**

Go through the list again and ask your child to estimate how much time she expects each assignment to take. Pad the time when possible. The skill of learning to estimate time is difficult; don't expect the estimates to be accurate. It's okay to suggest an alternative, but it's not critical that time estimates be right—yet. That will develop over time and practice.

3 **Prioritize and Plan**

You want to teach her to think about what is most important and why. Let your child choose whether she wants to prioritize by high-medium-low or A-B-C (or something else, as long as it's clear). It's not as important that she be right as it is that she starts learning to ask the question. As she gets older, she'll add nuance (e.g., "That's due tomorrow, but I'm making it a medium priority because I can do it with my friends during break tomorrow").

Work together to order the homework. Number the assignments, starting with 1 for what she'll do first. Make the numbers large and circle them so they are really visible.

Plan breaks. Make sure she's not doing anything for more than about 20 minutes without some kind of a break, even if it's just standing and stretching.

**4 Monitor**

Once she gets started on her homework, she can use a stopwatch to get a sense of how long things take and to keep her breaks reasonable. As soon as possible, let her start monitoring herself, instead of doing it for her.

Remember that she probably won't follow the plan exactly. Once she starts, she may decide to get the math out of the way, or to take a break from reading. That's okay. As Eisenhower said, "Plans are useless, but planning is indispensable." What's important is that she takes the time to think it through and is learning to organize herself.

Over time, ask her what she is learning about how she learns. Is she noticing that it's harder for her to get the reading done if she puts it too far down on the list? Or that reading is like a break for her, so it should go after she does something really hard? This process not only helps the work get done more efficiently, but it is teaching your child to think about how she operates best, a self-awareness that is essential for self-management.

## Calendarize+

Using a calendar may seem like a general organization strategy for everyone, and one that isn't special for people with ADHD. But for people with ADHD, learning to use a calendar effectively can make the difference between success and failure. Unfortunately, getting kids with ADHD to learn to use a calendar can be incredibly difficult. Honestly, it took one of our daughters over three years to start using a calendar of any kind, and that was with a lot of focus and effort. Frankly, she found it completely overwhelming.

For people who struggle with planning, motor coordination challenges, or decision making, using a calendar can be quite stressful. Sure, it's useful. But the mechanics of using it can be difficult for our kids (or ourselves). Whether you are using a paper calendar, a whiteboard, or a digital version, data entry is tedious—and so is stopping whatever you're doing to remember to add something to

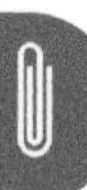

a calendar. Oftentimes, it takes some success over time for kids to overcome the obstacles and feel motivated to use a calendar.

Calendarize+ goes a step beyond just using a calendar. To "calendarize" means to capture your to-do's and include them on your calendar—to take everything that needs to get done and make sure it's captured with a time associated with it. When we actively schedule time to do something, we're more likely to get it done. For younger kids, you might use a big whiteboard in the kitchen, and for older kids you might move to a digital system that the whole family uses. Whenever you start, it's a terrific skill for our kids to learn.

So when your child says, "I want to read that new book I got for my birthday," you might ask, "When? Would you like to put some time on the calendar this weekend for you to do some reading?" Now, your son might look at you like you have 10 heads, but you've planted a seed—you've begun to teach him that it helps to plan a time to do something that he wants to do.

It also helps to remember that, these days, calendars are usually linked to reminder systems, alarms, and other bells and whistles to improve organization. To use a calendar effectively means learning to set alarms, be part of groups, consider what's on other people's calendars, and more. Calendarize+ is a process you can't start too early for kids with ADHD.

## Weekend Whiteboard

This strategy is a modified version of one taught by time-management educator Marydee Sklar. She suggests placing a large whiteboard on an easel in a high-traffic area like the kitchen prior to the start of the weekend (on Thursday evening, for example). On the whiteboard, each family member lists his or her chores and homework assignments that need to get done over the weekend, plus things they want to do over the weekend (such as play a family game or get together with friends). You can use a single color, or color-code the entries per family member if that's helpful or fun for everyone and doesn't add any stress.

At the regularly agreed-upon time (perhaps Friday before dinner), work on the whiteboard together as a family. Write "Saturday" and "Sunday" in large letters at the top, and wipe and rewrite the items to arrange them under the day the task is planned to get done. During this process, estimate together how long each thing will take. In some cases, decide specifically when something will get done. For example, you might agree: "Saturday, you can watch a half-hour of cartoons, then we'll all clean the bathrooms and kitchen. Then, after lunch, we'll all go play Frisbee in the park. Because you don't have too much homework, you can wait until Sunday afternoon to do it."

Make sure the whiteboard includes some play items. However, if some of those things need to get postponed for another weekend, that's fine—just remember to help your family understand why and assure them that you haven't forgotten. Writing a play item on the white board is not a promise; it's just a great way for your kids (and spouse) to communicate what they'd like to see happen. The weekend whiteboard is a great way to get a sense of what types of activities motivate your child.

With a weekend whiteboard, you are a lot less likely to get to Sunday night wondering where the weekend went. You might not get everything done, but there's a much stronger likelihood that the essential things—the ones staring you in the face in big, bold letters—will get accomplished.

## Mind Mapping

Mind mapping, or creating a mind map (a diagram that connects information in a visual format) is a simple, nonlinear organization strategy that can be useful to the ADHD brain. For someone with ADHD, this process is often more comfortable than creating a linear outline. Think of it as a tree with a central trunk (the central theme or idea) and many branches and limbs (related or even non-related ideas). Some branches and limbs connect with each other.

If many different topics are going on in your child's brain at once, mind mapping makes it easier for her to capture her thoughts and information. The same is true when bouncing back and forth between different ideas, as you might during brainstorming. It also helps someone who is challenged by working memory to visualize information.

A mind map can include words, images, numbers, and colors to make it more fun to create and the information easier to remember. According to research, the combination of words and pictures is six times better for remembering information than words alone.

Mind maps can be used to flesh out new ideas or outline a project or to help a child reinforce what she is learning in a class. This activity can help kids find the connections and links between different ideas. It can be useful for planning complex tasks, like a research project, or mundane tasks, like cleaning the kitchen after dinner. It can also be used to think through ideas or plan events or activities.

To get started mind mapping, pick something fun, like a sleepover party. On a clean sheet of paper, your child can either draw or write *sleepover party.* If she'd like to, she can put the main idea in a box, circle, bubble, or whatever shape she likes. Then help her identify the key things that will be involved as branches leading out from sleepover. The branches might be *food*, *where to sleep*, *when*, *guest list*, *what to play*, and *what to watch*.

Each of those branches then can branch off into limbs that correspond to those ideas. For example, next to *guest list*, she might draw arrows or lines pointing to the names of friends she wants to invite. In the area of *when*, she might draw arrows pointing to options for the date and time. That might get her thinking she wants to ask a certain friend: when would be a good time for her? She can go back to the guest list and highlight that friend's name and connect it to another line that says "call to choose a date." Continue this process until she gets all of her ideas for the sleepover party out on the single piece of paper. She can then create another mind map for planning the activities or food.

There is a lot of room for individual expression in a mind map—there's no right or wrong way to do it. What's most important is that it can give your child a process for managing and organizing information in a way that is better suited for the way her brain is wired, with the added bonus of unleashing her creativity.

## Build In Processing Time

Some kids with ADHD have a difficult time processing information on short notice. They often struggle with processing speed, memory recall, and even anxiety. They need time to think about things and can get incredibly frustrated if they are asked to produce ideas, information, or schoolwork on short notice.

In school, children who have difficulty initiating tasks may be challenged by blank-page paralysis. They may start to freak out or shut down when given an open-ended assignment. They don't know where to start, and they haven't had a chance to think it through. It is stressful when a teacher says, "You may begin. You have 30 minutes." These kids also struggle with processing information or requests from parents. A simple question like "What do you want to do this weekend?" may be met with blank stares and even tears. If an immediate answer is expected, the child will likely respond, "I don't know." A day or two later, she may come back to you with ideas, but by that point, you have probably already made arrangements for the weekend.

Sometimes, we need to give kids time to think about things, to noodle over them in the back of their minds. Allowing extra time to process information aids in organization, improves attention, and reduces emotional intensity. This isn't about giving them an extra five minutes or a few hours. This is communicating with your child about something that requires his attention a full day or two in advance. He needs to roll it around in his mind's eye, try it on, and get comfortable with it.

For younger kids, this means giving them a writing prompt or topic the day before they are expected to do an in-class writing assignment. For older kids, it may mean working with them to make sure they choose a theme for their term paper early on so that they don't spend all semester choosing a topic. When it comes to personal matters, it helps to introduce ideas to your kids, let them be for a day or two, and then circle back by bringing up the conversation again. Little by little, you can encourage your child to consider ideas without adding the stress of demanding an immediate response.

It might take a week to get through a conversation with your son about what he wants to do this summer. But when you do this, you'll be teaching him to think through the matter before making a decision. There is also a stronger likelihood he'll buy-in to whatever summer arrangements are made.

Giving kids extra time to process information helps them learn to become decision makers in their own lives. As they grow up, they are going to have to make many decisions, both large and small. If you start now by giving them time to practice, they will learn to make decisions more quickly over time.

## Identify High-Productivity Time

Effort management is an aspect of executive function that is not well understood, but getting a handle on it can be helpful for understanding and managing a child's ADHD. Most people have a rhythm to their lives—there are early birds who feel productive in the wee hours of the day, and night owls who feel more productive later in the day. This doesn't necessarily hold true for ADHD, as one of its markers is inconsistency.

With ADHD, there are good days and bad days; sometimes a person with ADHD is on, and sometimes that person is off. There is no rhyme or reason—it's just that sometimes the brain is hitting the target, and sometimes it's misfiring. This inconsistency can be frustrating for the child with ADHD as well as for those who aren't sure what they can rely on. A teacher might report that a kid with ADHD is doing great one week and can't understand why things seem to be falling apart the next.

You can't plan for all of the inconsistencies of the ADHD brain, but you can maximize effectiveness by identifying times that tend to be more highly productive than others. You can help your child learn to pay attention and to begin to notice her typical high points and low points in a day. Sometimes, she may feel high or low in response to a certain teacher or activity, or her rhythm is dictating her energy level. Map this out as best as you can to identify and then maximize high-productivity time.

For example, if you know your child is usually productive in the morning, advocate for having his most difficult classes scheduled for the mornings and plan weekend homework for Saturday or Sunday mornings. If she typically gets tired after lunch, that's a great time for a class that she finds interesting or that doesn't require a lot of effort. For younger kids, it can also be a good time for a nap. You'll also know that after lunch is *not* a great time to ask her to clean her room or be extra nice to her little sister.

## The Portable Homework Toolbox

Creating a portable homework toolbox—a file storage box with all the homework supplies a child is likely to need—adds organization and novelty to the strategy "Flexible Homework Stations and Times" on page 71.

Purchase a file storage box with a lid and handle. Place a few hanging file folders inside. If possible, use color-coded file folders for different classes or subjects. Add other items that tend to be used during homework sessions. Tape and glue, markers and pencils, erasers, rulers, and construction paper are great for younger kids. For older students, include a calculator, pens, lined paper, a dictionary/thesaurus, a protractor, a ruler, and other items specific to your child's courses. For example, a chemistry student might need the Periodic Table of Elements; a literature student might need a pocket guide to Shakespeare.

Work with your child to develop his personal portable homework toolbox, instead of just doing it for him. For a younger kid, you can ask what he thinks should be included, but put it together in an organized fashion if he doesn't seem interested in doing it himself. As your kid gets older, help him develop the list (or mind map; see page 102) of what should be included, and work together to develop the box. Creating the toolbox together will help your child think in terms of planning for supplies. Ideally, by the time he goes off to college, he won't want to leave home without it!

## School Paper Management

On the one hand, kids have a tendency to lose things and don't always understand what's important, so we don't want them to throw away something they're going to need later in the semester (like a test to use for studying for an exam). On the other hand, kids have a tendency to be pack rats, and we want to teach them to throw things out and learn to save what's important.

Teach your child to save everything throughout the school quarter or semester (or, for older students, for the entire school year). Add some structure to the process, whether by using file folders, a binder, or an accordion file for each class or subject. Encourage your child to file away her papers every weekend. Emphasize the importance of saving everything until the end of a term or the school year. That way, she'll have quizzes and tests to use as study aids for exams, and she'll understand that the information she's learning can be cumulative.

Once your child is done with the work for that term or school year, help her determine what she wants to do with those papers. Sort through everything and let her choose what she wants to save. Saved papers can be stored in a memory box, if that sounds good to her. She might want to throw all the papers out or even have a shredding party to celebrate her success. She might decide to save some material, like vocabulary words or language notes, for future reference.

You can start this process with very young children. It's a great way to teach them to begin to think about what is important and what's not. Shredding busywork, while saving special projects, helps your child learn to be discerning—and to appreciate the value of her own hard work. If she is inclined to throw everything away, make the effort to help her recognize what she did that was particularly valuable, so she can celebrate her accomplishments. If she is inclined to keep everything, make the effort to help her learn to part with papers that are no longer useful.

## Homework Insurance Policies

It's hard enough to help your child complete his homework, but then there's still a risk that it won't get turned in. It is not uncommon for kids with ADHD to forget to put their homework in their schoolbag, forget to turn it in, or lose it completely. When he's lucky, he finds it weeks later (when there's a 0 on the grading sheet) in the bottom of his schoolbag. When he's not so lucky, it's missing in action, and he will likely have to redo the homework assignment. Redoing work that's already been done is infuriating for everyone, and there are usually tears involved. It's more common than you might imagine.

You can ask for accommodations in the case of an Individualized Education Program (IEP) or a 504 Plan to increase the likelihood that homework will get turned in—once it's arrived in the classroom. But getting it from home to school is another challenge. Homework folders and other tactics can be helpful. You'll also want to minimize the risk of losing homework by taking out these insurance policies:

1. Take pictures of homework when it's completed. Smartphones make it easy to record your child's work. You can gamify this by doing a fun photo shoot, or just keep it practical. Consider it insurance against tomorrow night's meltdown.
2. Adopt the mantra: "Your homework's not done until it's put away." Say it every day (in a singsong voice without judgment) so that eventually, all you have to say is "Your homework's not done until . . . " and your child will say (while rolling his eyes, of course), "It's put away." The eye roll is worth it to help your child put the homework into the schoolbag before going to bed.
3. Set up a landing zone for your child (younger ones, especially) where school materials are placed as soon as he comes in the door after school. Also have a launchpad for completed items (such as his schoolbag) for finished homework so that they're ready for takeoff the next day. The landing zone and launchpad can be the same place if that makes sense in your house, but they don't have to be.

## Keep It Simple

Some common pitfalls when it comes to reward systems were covered in "Reassess Your Reward Strategy" on page 93. However, the greatest challenge is often that the system is just too complicated!

Having to keep track of stickers, checkmarks, and smiley faces can be tedious and time consuming. If we try to track too many things at once, well . . . that's a recipe for limited success and overall disappointment when our kids can't remember what's on the list. And what if we struggle with our own executive function challenges? It's hard enough to find our keys, so how are we going to remember to check off 26 items on a list every night?

Parents need solutions that can be implemented quickly and easily, both inside and outside the home. That means you need to keep it simple by focusing on only one behavior at a time. When we do that, there is a better chance we can help our kids focus clearly and see some success. When we expect a little less from our kids in terms of volume and expect them to do specific things a little better or a little more carefully, they tend to feel proud of their accomplishments. And as we've said, success breeds success.

Focusing on improving just one skill can be difficult when we have many concerns about our child and there are so many things we want them to accomplish. We want to make sure they're ready for adulthood—and even for kids as young as age seven, we start to feel as if we're running out of time. But we must remember that our kids' complex brains struggle to retain and process information. If we pile on too much and expect them to work on developing many different skills at once, they can start to feel disheartened and may be inclined to give up. So try to keep it simple. Limit your household rules to the essentials and try not to pile on too many chores. Allow your kids to do one thing at a time, let them feel good about it, and then move on to helping them improve the next skill.

That's the reality of your child's life. It can be difficult to manage. It can even be frustrating and scary and overwhelming, but you now have a whole arsenal of strategies and techniques at your fingertips. As you continue your journey and try out the ideas suggested, keep the following in mind.

## Avoiding Crises

ADHD is a manageable condition. As you begin to understand it better, you can learn strategies for managing it more effectively. And as you do that, you will teach your child to understand himself better, without shame or embarrassment, and learn to take conscious steps to improve his self-management—which is key to his long-term independence and success.

We hope that this book helps you see that all of the challenging issues that accompany ADHD can be addressed and eventually overcome . . . with time, patience, some strategic problem solving, and intentional, thoughtful, conscious parenting.

When you are overly worried, hovering, and afraid to let your child learn from mistakes, it makes it difficult for him to find the confidence he needs to overcome and live well with this condition—a condition that causes him to make more mistakes than his peers. On the other hand, when you are understanding and knowledgeable, accepting and strategic, you make it possible for your child to learn resilience, which research teaches us is more important to long-term success than intelligence or environment. Resiliency is one of the most important skills to cultivate for success in adult life. In this book, we've introduced a wide variety of tactics, strategies, and concepts to help you foster that resilience in your child and your family as a whole.

## Asking for Help

In different ways throughout this book, we've talked about the importance of teaching your child to ask for and accept the help he needs. Asking for help is a critical component to ADHD management, and it starts with you.

Many of us suffer from "superparent" disease. We feel like we should be able to do it all ourselves, whatever it may be. Worse, we are sure that it's just easier if we do it ourselves. This tends to set us up for exhaustion and frustration. We try to do everything ourselves so that we don't bother anyone, or we grow increasingly resentful as we start to feel put upon.

Asking for help is a great leadership skill, and it's an essential one for parents to master and model. When we ask for help we:

1. Give others an opportunity to take responsibility
2. Let go of control
3. Teach our kids the value of self-advocacy

Each of those themes surfaces repeatedly throughout this book. They are absolutely critical to your success as a parent when your goal is to help your child learn self-management.

Sometimes we get caught up in the details of our lives, and we think that our job is to help our child finish an assignment, follow directions, or do what is expected of her. That may be true in the moment. But the truth is, our job as parents is much bigger than that. Ultimately, our job is to raise our children to be able to function independently when they become adults—to know themselves, understand their strengths and challenges, and feel confident in problem solving and making thoughtful decisions.

When kids have ADHD, our job is to teach them, step by step, what is required to be in charge of themselves and their beautiful, complicated brains. To do that effectively, they are going to need to learn that asking for help is not a sign of weakness; in fact, it is a sign of strength. Whether we're teaching them to ask a teacher to work with them to chunk down a semester-long research project or to advocate for accommodations for learning challenges in college (which they must do on their own), their success, at least in part, depends on their ability to ask for and accept help.

## What to Expect as Your Child Ages

Expect things to change. As your child matures, you'll notice that the way that ADHD presents will likely shift over time. A hyperactive young kid will eventually learn to manage the physical need for activity, but he may struggle more with mental hyperactivity that keeps him awake at night. A chatty third grader who tells his mother everything after school might want to spend a lot of time texting with friends in high school, debriefing the social dynamics of the day.

Transition times, in particular, are likely to cause some stress and tension. While kids are making progress in some areas, you may notice slight regression in other areas. That's normal and generally no cause for alarm. They are trying to get a handle on many different aspects of self-management, and when they are focusing on one thing, they may temporarily lose focus on another. A child who finally learned to unpack his lunchbox each day at the end of middle school may forget when high school calls upon him to focus on so many other organizational skills. A few weeks into school, he will probably regain the skill (if reminded), but a temporary lapse is not cause for concern.

Truly, it takes years for all kids to integrate everything they're learning and begin to feel like they've really got it together. Generally, it takes longer for kids with ADHD. So be patient with the process, and remember that, in general, the rational part of the brain is not fully developed until at least age 25. It is reasonable to expect that you will provide appropriate scaffolding throughout their high school years and into their early adulthood, reconnecting to your own sources of support as necessary to help you provide the support your child needs.

Many parents return to our group coaching programs, for example, when their teens enter their junior year of high school, which in the United States tends to be the most difficult year for most kids. These parents have been doing quite well with their teens for years, but when the added stressors of upcoming transition come into play, the communication with their kids needs to be different, and parents find they need a tune-up. There's no shame in this—it's to be expected.

So the bottom line of parenting ADHD over time is the same message Elaine learned and taught when she was teaching pregnancy yoga classes: Expect the unexpected, and be prepared for anything.

## The Most Important Message

If we boil it all down to the most important lesson in this book, it's this: Don't try to do it alone. In an article, "ADHD Diagnosis: The Good, the Bad and the Parent's Role," Dr. Edward M. Hallowell writes, "It is true that people with ADHD tend to contribute to the world in a very positive way. But first, they must get a handle on what's going on. And they cannot do it alone." He continues, applying that message specifically to parents: "The most important thing for parents to do when their children have ADHD is to find the support you need, and use it! Get parent training that will help you understand your child's experience, so that you're able to help your child more effectively learn to self-manage. Join support groups or coaching groups so that you don't hold the frustrations inside. Tell trusted others about what you're up against. As you get the training and support you need, for your child and yourself, you'll have the skills and the strength to persevere. And you'll be teaching your child the valuable lesson of reaching out for help and support. You cannot do it alone, nor should you try."

According to Andrea Bilbow, a British advocate and educator honored by Queen Elizabeth II for her work on behalf of families living with ADHD, there is "one common denominator that stands behind every child's success: a mother (or dad) who has been an incredible advocate for her child." Effective advocacy is a whole lot easier when you find partners for support.

When you have a child with ADHD, in all likelihood, you will be actively parenting a bit longer than typical parents. There's nothing wrong with that—it just is what it is. So pace yourself for the long haul. Give things time to change. Take advantage of the strategies offered in this book. And don't stop here. We want to encourage you to take things to the next level. Find a support structure to help you take what you've learned in this book and put it into action. That's where the rubber meets the road. And that's where you will find the kind of transformational change you're really looking for.

Whether you get help from us online and on the phone, from a local support group, from a coach or a therapist, or from some combination, remember that we are stronger together than any of us are on our own. At ImpactADHD, we are passionate about the importance of parents understanding the challenges children with ADHD are facing, getting clear about the specific changes you want to achieve, and finding the most effective path to get there.

The more you identify the challenges your kid faces and help her learn to manage them consciously, the more likely she will find success overcoming or learning to live with her challenges as an adult. Like any other neurological medical condition, ADHD can and should be approached consciously for an excellent quality of life.

So as we bring this book of fun and functional strategies to a close, we want to acknowledge you for doing this work, for making it this far, and for investing your time and energy in learning about how to best support your children. We know it's not easy, and just getting through a book like this can be a challenge! But we also know that it is well worth your effort—for you, your child with ADHD, and your whole family.

And we want to encourage you to keep it going!

Take some time to explore the Resources section on page 152. Find the guidance that works for you, something that offers you structure and accountability, and fosters calm and confidence. Keep teaching your child to understand and manage himself, and keep modeling for him the incredible value of asking for help.

Get the support you need to slowly but surely teach your child to ask for and accept help. No one has to do it alone. That is the true secret to creating the future your family deserves.

## APPENDIX

# School-Specific Strategies

Most of the strategies included in this book are designed for you to use with your children at home. Yet no book of strategies for managing ADHD would be complete without attention to how it presents at school. After all, we know that many of you are advocating around these same challenges for your child during the day.

What follows is a list of the strategies from the book that are also particularly useful at school. Then, we provide some strategies that are specific to the school environment. While some of these may also be useful at home, their primary effectiveness is in the school environment.

## At-Home Strategies to Use in School

### ATTENTION

- Get Moving (page 46)
- Medication (page 48)
- Identify Motivators (page 48)
- Assess Your Child's Noise Tolerance (page 53)
- Minimize Distractions (page 55)
- Get Attention Before Giving Direction (page 56)

### HYPERACTIVITY

- Calm the Brain with Physical Activity (page 63)
- Allow Your Child to Not Be Still (page 64)
- Give 'em a Job (page 64)
- Target Physical Activity Before and During Brainwork (page 65)
- Fidget to Focus (page 67)
- Become a Scribe (page 67)
- Gamify Routine Tasks and Chores (see page 70)

### IMPULSIVITY

- Brain Breaks (page 80)
- Celebrate Being Good (page 82)
- Token Economy (page 83)
- Code Words (page 88)

### ORGANIZATION

- Token Economy (page 83)
- Keep Things Visual (page 94)
- Prepare for Transitions (page 95)
- Keep It Simple (page 109)
- Mind Mapping (page 102)
- Build In Processing Time (page 104)

### EMOTIONALITY

- Make Mistakes Matter of Fact (page 124)
- Speed Up by Slowing Down (page 130)
- Ask About Challenges (page 134)

## Strategies for the School Environment

The best tool for managing ADHD at school is an open relationship with your child's teacher(s), where you can share what works at home, and your child's teacher can share strategies she's uncovered that may work at school. In addition, the following are some strategies and tactics that are specific to the school environment.

### WORD MIRRORING

This is a strategy to support kids who struggle with impulsivity and have a difficult time paying attention to something from start to finish. They are easily distracted and tend to respond to anything they find stimulating instead of holding their focus on what they are doing. Word mirroring is a trick from the world of improvisational comedy that can help a lot with this issue.

To word-mirror, children are consciously thinking about the words that someone else is saying at the very instant that they are hearing the words. They should actually repeat the words to themselves *in their heads, but not speak them out loud.* When you try it, you'll notice that you're a split second behind the person speaking, but you can really keep up with what she's saying, and what she's saying keeps your attention. It's difficult to get distracted when you are word-mirroring.

When kids are listening to their teachers for content or the steps for directions, word mirroring can help them stay on top of what is expected of them. Not only will they be paying closer attention, but also the process of repeating the words silently in their heads reaches another portion of the brains, and that increases the likelihood of remembering.

### THINK OF A QUESTION

This is a strategy to support kids who struggle with interrupting, specifically kids who interrupt in class because they are struggling to pay attention or because they are making connections in their own brains that are leading to further questions. In this case, they have a tendency to blurt out questions (or answers) to keep themselves engaged or to help themselves make sense of the directions or the conversation.

If you think about it, overactive participation in the classroom (or at the dinner table) stems from an enthusiastic desire to be involved. That's a good thing. Most of us would rather have our kids *want* to be involved than to check out and not care.

Our goal in these situations is to teach them *how* to be involved productively instead of coming down on them for exuberant engagement (which is often the message they are receiving). They need to know that you and their teachers understand that they are not intentionally causing distractions to annoy other students, teachers, siblings, and even parents.

Teach your child to think of questions to ask while he is listening to others' conversations or to directions—as many questions as possible. Help him focus on his curiosity. He can write the questions down or hold them in his head (depending on the strength of his working memory). The goal is not to ask them out loud but to collect them as he listens all the way through. Help him see that thinking up questions is a great strategy for him to stay engaged. Over time, you can teach him to notice how many of his questions are answered by the end of the directions or conversation.

## STICKY NOTE PATIENCE

This strategy supports kids who struggle with interrupting, either because they are afraid they won't remember or because it keeps them engaged in what is going on. It's a great companion to the "Think of a Question" strategy above.

First, help your child understand the source of his interruptions. Does he struggle with remembering things? Does he tend to want to have his questions addressed right away? Help him see that, the way his brain is wired, it's normal for him to want to address his thoughts right away but that sometimes it's important to learn to hold your thoughts or questions until someone else is finished. Like taking turns when playing a game, it's a skill he needs to practice and learn to master. Then ask him if he wants to learn a strategy to help him learn how.

Have your child put a small stack of sticky notes and a pen/pencil on his desk at the beginning of every class. (You can practice at the dinner table, too.) Encourage your child to write down any comments, thoughts, or questions that are distracting him from paying attention to the lesson, the directions, or the conversation. He can capture anything that comes to his mind or even doodle on the paper when he needs a fidget.

The sticky note becomes a reminder that he is working on not interrupting and is awaiting his turn to talk. He may find, at the end, that he's captured an idea that would be a good topic for a writing assignment or that all of his questions were eventually answered. Most of all, it brings awareness to this process for him and gives him a strategy to help him learn to manage his desire to interrupt over time.

## Accommodations for Exams and Tests: Specialized Testing

Kids who struggle with impulsivity often have trouble with test taking and other methods used by schools to determine what a child has learned. Sometimes, their memory takes a break, and no matter how well prepared they are, they cannot retrieve the information. Other times, they are so distracted by other kids that they cannot concentrate on the task at hand. Their impulses lead them to stand up, walk around, let their attention jump around on the page, and/or misread the questions—all in an effort to try to organize their brains.

These accommodations can help your child demonstrate what she is learning in school by limiting distractions and other things that trigger impulsive behaviors:

- **Oral exams.** Ask to have your child tested verbally so that she can demonstrate her understanding of the material, and get clarification on questions that she may be too impulsive to read properly.
- **Scribes.** Ask to have someone write for your child when there are long answers or short essays involved. Even writing out sentences for vocabulary words can help.

- **Private rooms for testing.** Ask to have your child placed in a private room for taking tests. During standardized tests, there is often a small room with other children that is less distracting, and offers more breaks and extra time.

## Chunk It Down

*Chunking* is a term for breaking large amounts of information into chunks that the brain can handle effectively. An average brain can hold about seven pieces of information before it gets overwhelmed. Social security, credit card, and telephone numbers are all chunked. Consider the number 2135559409. As a 10-digit number, it's overwhelming. But when chunked into 213-555-9409, it's easily recognized and much easier to memorize as a telephone number.

Children with ADHD often get overwhelmed long before they get to seven pieces of information. They will eventually get to that capacity, but when working memory is compromised, it will take them longer than their same-age peers.

Chunking is particularly effective for kids with ADHD who struggle with organization because it breaks complex information into parts that are easier to manage. A book report may feel overwhelming, but it seems more manageable when the steps are clearly identified, and put into a sequence: (1) Read the book (one chapter at a time), (2) write down notes about what you liked about it, (3) write a thesis statement, (4) write the details, and (5) write a conclusion. Once the information is chunked, a child can be directed to focus on only one item at a time. It helps her avoid feeling too anxious, as she has only the one task to accomplish. It also helps her feel clear on the one item that requires her attention.

In addition to chunking down schoolwork, you can also break down the steps of household chores. Instead of asking your daughter to clean her room, you can ask her to put the clothes in the hamper. Once that is completed, you can work together to identify the next task, and the next.

## Make Some Unusual Requests in IEPs and 504 Plans

There are many terrific resources to help you determine what to request in your child's IEPs and 504 Plans, and we encourage you to investigate the Resources section on page 152 for more on that. You can't go wrong with standard requests like extra time.

We also want to encourage you to get creative when asking for support. Think about what really helps your child be successful, and remember to ask your child for guidance. You may discover that there are some simple accommodations that can have a dramatic impact. For example, a calming kit toolbox (see page 121) at school might be powerfully effective for a child who is struggling with emotional management, or making your child the "attendance runner" every morning can help a hyperactive child transition into his day.

One of our children loves math but struggles with reading, so she was allowed to keep sudoku worksheets in the classroom to calm her down when she would get stressed out. So ask for peer mentors and additional check-ins from teachers or paraprofessionals, as well as other strategies to make sure your child feels supported and not isolated at school. You may not get everything you ask for, but one thing is certain: If you don't ask, you're not likely to get something that could make or break your child's school year.

## Permit Use of Technology

Many of our children, even young ones in elementary school, have access to technology in school. Even if that type of technology is a little foreign to us, we want to help our kids use everything at their disposal to maximize their success.

As a parent, particularly with children younger than high school age, request that all assignments, homework, test dates, handouts, and so forth, be available online, whether it's via a class website or a schoolwide portal. For you to effectively scaffold your child's success in school, you have to be able to know what is expected of her for each teacher, and by when.

Also request an accommodation to allow your child to use her own technology in class, as appropriate. For example, if your child has a phone or an iPad with a camera, you might want to ask for an accommodation to allow her to use it in class to take a photo of notes or assignments during the school day and/or to take a picture of the blackboard to capture her homework assignments. If appropriate, she could also use this technology to send herself message reminders or add tasks to her digital calendar.

It is fine to include conditions so that she does not abuse the privilege or taunt other children with it. If it is handled well and the communication is clear, then technology offers enhanced opportunities for organization that should not be ignored just because it is not available to everyone. Dismiss any arguments that it's not fair to the other children, and learn about your child's rights to an education that works for her.

## Systems for Moving Information to and from School

For every child, at every age, you want to make sure they have a clear system in place for transferring information, assignments, and completed work to and from school. It's not important that it be a single system—in fact, it's unlikely that one system will work for all children, or even that one child will use the same system every year. As classes and school expectations change, the system will change with it.

But be clear: Every child with ADHD needs to understand the agreed-upon system to transfer work between home and school. Some schools or teachers will require binders, while others will prefer individual notebooks for each class. Some teachers will have a homework notebook, and others will use an accordion file.

What's most important is to figure out what works for your child, on a year-by-year basis. Don't hesitate to ask for a single binder if you know that individual notebooks are more likely to get lost, and don't hesitate to ask for an accordion file if you know your child needs to put everything in one place. Most schools have a default system for management. If it's not a good fit for your child, advocate for something that is.

## Educating Educators

Most teachers have to be jacks-of-all-trades, so they may know a little about a lot of things. Certainly, you know your child better than they do. You may find it frustrating that your child's teacher does not possess all the knowledge about ADHD that you have. Although teachers are becoming more knowledgeable about this complicated problem, the progress is happening slowly. In the meantime, the more compassion you bring to your child's teacher, the better it will be for everyone.

Although you want to encourage your child's teachers to learn more about ADHD, start by asking them if they are open to you sharing resources with them. Explain that you know they are really busy and that it's challenging to have children with ADHD in their classes, so you'd like to be able to support them however possible. Consider buying them a teacher's membership to CHADD, or talking to your school principal or counselor about bringing CHADD's Teacher to Teacher program into your school. Offer to bring in targeted articles or information when you think it would be especially useful. Come from a place of service, instead of demanding support.

When you do, you'll be in a better position to ask more of your child's specific teachers. Help them understand that accommodations they make for children with ADHD will benefit the entire class. For example, whenever possible, ask them to connect their lessons to real-life circumstances, illustrating relevance and helping children connect to the information. Encourage teachers to give succinct instructions, and repeat them slowly. Ask them to call out what's important for the entire class. By saying, "You need to write this down, this is important, these are the three things you need to remember," all children in the class will benefit, and your child will not feel singled out.

Help your child's teachers understand that all kids' brains will take a break to process information, whether it's scheduled or not, so encourage them to give water breaks, snack breaks, and especially physical breaks! One of our child's teachers actually gave 10-minute fresh-air breaks every day in fourth grade, and it was great for the whole class.

## Advocate for Social Thinking Curricula

Advocate for your child's school to bring in programs that formally enhance social skills and self-awareness in the school environment. There are literally hundreds of antibullying, mindfulness, social skills, positive classroom, and other kinds of curricula available to educators who are interested in improving social dynamics.

For example, many school districts are beginning to incorporate Congressional Award–winning speech-language pathologist Michelle Garcia Winner's practices into their daily curriculum. Michelle Garcia Winner does a lot of training with multiple modalities for all age levels on what is expected behavior and what is considered unexpected behavior for any individual in a particular situation. In her visuals for younger kids, expected behavior appears as a blue thought, and unexpected behavior appears as a red thought. She has many worksheets, storyboards, and comic books that help kids practice social thinking. The materials help remind them of what to do or how to work through things when they get in a situation they are unsure of. More information on Michelle Garcia Winner's practices can be found in the Resources section on page 152.

You do not have to be an expert on these curricula or be able to recommend a specific program. First, try to get the ball rolling to raise awareness. Offer support to the administration to help make it happen. Perhaps you can serve on a committee to investigate programs for the administration to consider. Your interest in promoting something that will serve the entire community will help the school see you as an ally and enhance your ability to advocate for your child.

# Resources

## ImpactADHD

ImpactADHD provides vital support, solutions, and structures for parents who want to help their kids with ADHD reach their full potential. Using a combination of training, coaching, and support, ImpactADHD provides a practical how-to approach, whether parents are new to the world of complex kids or worn-out from years of management. By helping parents put strategies into action and coaching them to make those strategies work best for their families, ImpactADHD guides parents to radically improve family life and empower their kids for independence and success. Everything at ImpactADHD was developed to provide support for parents that is effective, affordable, and accessible to all—online and on the phone.

**Award-Winning Blog and Free Support:** Developed as a targeted resource exclusively for parents of children with ADHD and related challenges, ImpactADHD's award-winning blog offers hundreds of original tips, articles, guest expert articles, and vetted resources for parents, all free of charge. We invite any parent of a complex child to sign up for our weekly newsletter, which includes links to the week's newest articles. Monthly webinars and other free training events are offered throughout the year. Currently, parents from 180 countries around the world use the free resources available on ImpactADHD.com. **(ImpactADHD.com /newsletter-signup/)**

**Videos, Trainings, and Programs:** Through a range of videos, online home-study programs, live online trainings, and group and individual coaching (on the phone), ImpactADHD provides parents with behavior therapy and management support to reduce parent stress, strengthen parent confidence, and improve outcomes for children with ADHD. All programs are interactive, combining some element of coaching, training, and support to improve participation and achieve results. **(ImpactADHD.com/how-we-can-help/parenting-programs/)**

**Serving the ADHD Community:** At ImpactADHD, we speak for the parents of children with ADHD and all the related coexisting conditions that tend to accompany it. In collaboration with other professionals, ImpactADHD consistently sheds light on the importance of the parenting experience in effective management of ADHD, enhancing awareness in the larger ADHD community. Other professionals are invited to join us in this important work as guest experts and affiliates. **(ImpactADHD.com/our-team/affiliates/)**

**Summary of Resources for Parents:** While there are more resources to support families with ADHD than we could ever capture, we do publish an incredible resource section on ImpactADHD.com, vetted from input from parents in our community, which includes Recommended Reading and Useful Tools.

## Websites

This section highlights some of our favorite websites, but for a more thorough list, we encourage you to visit ImpactADHD.com. Some of these resources are products available for purchase, and others are offered free of charge, but each one shares guidance and specific tips to support you on this journey.

## NONPROFIT ORGANIZATIONS

- Children and Adults with Attention-Deficit/Hyperactivity Disorder (search for information, and local support groups and professionals): CHADD.org
- Understood.org
- Attention Deficit Disorder Association (ADDA): ADD.org
- ADHD Coaches Organization: ADHDcoaches.org

## GENERAL WEBSITES FOR ADHD

- Help4ADHD.org (National Resource Center on ADHD, funded by the CDC and a project of CHADD—also has a helpline)
- ADDitudemag.com
- DrHallowell.com
- TotallyADD.com

## SUPPORT FOR CHILDREN AND TEENS

- ADHDkidsrock.com (kids blog about ADHD)
- BeyondBooksmart.com (executive function tutoring)
- EdgeFoundation.org (ADHD coaching for students)
- HeyYouADHD.com (young children)

## OTHER HELPFUL WEBSITES FOR PARENTS

- AttentionTalkRadio.com (hundreds of interviews with the world's leading experts)
- ADHDMarriage.com (seminar on ADHD and Marriage with Melissa Orlov)
- KidsintheHouse.com (video warehouse)
- LearningWorksforKids.com (apps and games recommendations)
- ADDClasses.com
- Mindmapping.com
- SocialThinking.com

### IMPACTADHD PROGRAMS AND SUPPORT FOR PARENTS AND FAMILIES

- ADHDParentManual.com
- SanitySchool.com
- HomeworkHeadaches.net
- MinimizeMeltdowns.com
- ParentSuccessSystem.com

### IMPACTADHD NEWSLETTER (IMPACTADHD.COM/NEWSLETTER-SIGNUP/) VIDEOS FOR MANAGING ADHD (FOR ADULTS AND/OR CHILDREN)

- ParentingWithImpact.com
- ADDCrusher.com
- BeyondFocused.com
- TotallyADD.com

### SUPPORT GROUPS AND PROGRAMS FOR WOMEN WITH ADULT ADHD

- ADDConsults.com
- ADDiva.net
- ImpactADHD.com
- SariSolden.com

## Books

There are thousands of books about ADHD on the market, and it can be difficult for parents to know where to start. For a targeted, vetted recommended reading list and brief reviews, we encourage you to visit the book carousel on our website at ImpactADHD.com/Recommended-Reading/. Books are divided into the following categories: ADHD strategies; ADHD, learning disabilities, and mental health resources; general parenting; self-care; coaching/life lessons; relationships and marriage; health; and inspiration. Some of our favorite books include the following:

Barkley, Russell. *Taking Charge of ADHD: The Complete, Authoritative Guide for Parents.* New York: Guilford Press, 2013.

Bertin, Mark. *Mindful Parenting for ADHD: A Guide to Cultivating Calm, Reducing Stress, and Helping Children Thrive.* Oakland, CA: New Harbinger Publications, 2015.

Brown, Stuart, and Christopher Vaughan. *Play: How It Shapes the Brain, Opens the Imagination, and Invigorates the Soul.* New York: Avery, 2009.

Brown, Thomas E. *Attention Deficit Disorder: The Unfocused Mind in Children and Adults.* New Haven, CT: Yale University Press, 2006.

Brown, Thomas E. *Smart but Stuck: Emotions in Teens and Adults with ADHD.* San Francisco, CA: Jossey-Bass, 2014.

Dendy, Chris A. Zeigler. *Teaching Teens with ADD, ADHD & Executive Function Deficits: A Quick Reference Guide for Teachers and Parents. 2nd ed.* Bethesda, MD: Woodbine House, 2011.

Dorfman, Kelly. *Cure Your Child with Food: The Hidden Connection Between Nutrition and Childhood Ailments.* New York: Workman Publishing Company, 2013.

Dupar, Laurie. *Wacky Ways to Succeed with ADHD: The Never Before Fun, Creative Out-of-the Box Secrets That Will Get You Smiling and Surviving with ADHD.* Granite Bay, CA: Coaching for ADHD, 2015.

Hallowell, Edward M., and John J. Ratey. *Driven to Distraction (Revised): Recognizing and Coping with Attention Deficit Disorder.* New York: Anchor Books, 2011.

Matlen, Terry. *The Queen of Distraction: How Women with ADHD Can Conquer Chaos, Find Focus, and Get More Done.* Oakland, CA: New Harbinger Publications, 2014.

Orlov, Melissa. *The ADHD Effect on Marriage: Understand and Rebuild Your Relationship in Six Steps.* Fort Lauderdale, FL: Specialty Press/ADD Warehouse, 2010.